NATURE'S HEALING AGENTS

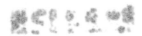

Other books by R. Swinburne Clymer, M.D.

Diet, The Way to Health
Race Regeneration
Making Health Certain
Your Health and Sanity

NATURE'S
HEALING AGENTS

THE MEDICINES OF NATURE
(or THE NATURA SYSTEM)

By

R. SWINBURNE CLYMER. M.D.

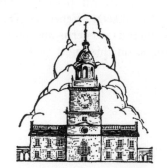

DORRANCE and COMPANY
Philadelphia

6 15 537

Cb2N

Author's Note

The dominant practice of medicine is known as the allopathic system. What may be generally termed as the opposite of this school is known as the homeopathic system. The early herbal system of practice became the Thomsonian system, and out of this emerged, or developed, the eclectic and later the physicomedical system. The Natura system of practice combined the agents considered most natural, as used by the Thomsonian, eclectic, and physiomedical systems, eschewing practically all poisons. The term *Natura* was preempted by patent No. 30,604, February 18, 1908 and used continually since then. Numerous concerns and publishers have infringed, and continue to infringe, on this right to the name for a system of practice.

NATURE, THE GREAT PHYSICIAN

Nature, the great physician, if permitted and not interfered with, will provide man's physical requirements. Sanitation will eliminate all impurities, so frequently the cause of disease. Nature and sanitation, given the opportunity, will prevent disease, or where it is present, help eliminate it.

The Natura Physician's Creed

The Natura physician is basically religious, spiritually inclined as were all physicians in times past who loved and lived for their profession. Their feelings are always with those who suffer, and their idea is to bring as much relief to the ill as may be in their power.

The Natura physician sees this statement in *Genesis* 1:29 as the Divine law for man's well-being.

This statement as a Divine edict is now more pertinent than ever in view of the late discoveries made by investigators, especially biochemists, interested in: What is life? What will offer greater life? What will sustain life? What will free man from illness brought about by his own disobedience to natural law?

The Statement of the Law

"And God said [the Law functioned], Behold, I have given you every herb bearing seed, which is upon the face of all the earth, and every tree, in which is the fruit of a tree yielding seed; to you it shall be for meat.*

"And to every beast of the earth, and to every fowl of the air, and to every thing that creepeth upon the earth, wherein there is life, I have given green herb for meat: and it was so."—*Genesis 1:29, 30.*

---

* i.e., food (Author's interpretation).

PROLOGUE

Until very recently, vegetables, cereals, and fruits were simply things to eat. In a way everyone, physician and layman, understood that these substances satisfied the appetite and at the same time supplied fuel to the body. Beyond this fact neither physician nor layman had much knowledge or were greatly concerned.

All this has changed. Bio-chemistry, instituted by Schuessler of Germany, discovered the fundamental fact that health and strength do not depend so much on the specific substances we ingest as food but on the vital organic and mineral contents of these substances.

When first cultivated the tomato was thought to be poisonous even by medical men of standing and was considered a cause of cancer and partaken of by few people. With its development into a large, luscious fruit-vegetable, the old idea was thrown into discard with many other erroneous popular opinions, and the tomato was accepted both as a wholesome food and as a delicacy. What is the real, though generally unknown, reason for its popularity? Nothing less than its richness in organic and mineral elements, possessing as it does an average of 82.50 potassium, 32.90 sodium, calcium, 29.40 phosphorus, besides other valuable elements, in each one thousand parts.

Swiss chard, once not even considered either herb or vegetable but a weed, is now almost as great a favorite as broccoli. Its contents per one thousand parts are: 62.70 sodium, 44.92 potassium, 21.69 calcium, 19.39 phosphorus, besides other elements just as valuable, though less in quantity.

Celery is possibly one of the most universally appreciated vegetables. Not so long ago it was considered an herb, splendid as a tea for the nervous. Celery, like the tomato and the apple, has developed from a favorite medicine into a food. Its contents per thousand parts are: 65.24 sodium, 48.60 potassium, 14.90 calcium, 14.49 phosphorus, and other elements, among which is chlorine, 17.80. Only one other vegetable is richer in this element. Tomatoes contain 18.00 per 1,000 parts.

Rhubarb is another vegetable that until recently was considered a medicine of value in constipation. Gradually it was accepted as good material for delicious pies, then as an appetizing sauce, and finally, splendid for the making of wine. Its contents per thousand parts are: 74.50 potassium, 12.55 calcium, 18.41 phosphorus, 6.80 chlorine, and other valued elements.

Lettuce, formerly good food for cattle and chickens, is now a universal favorite and is preparable in many forms. Its contents per thousand parts are 74.50 potassium, 26.56 calcium, 14.63 silicon, 13.82 chlorine, and other valued elements.

Beets once were cattle food, but due to their appearance and appeal to the appetite, gradually found their way to the table as food for man also. Their contents per thousand parts are 38.70 potassium, 9.00 chlorine, 9.00 sodium, and other elements.

Onions,[1] universally liked and as universally despised, are rich in potassium and phosphorus. They are the ideal remedy in the onset of colds and all bronchial trouble.

Snap beans (green) now on almost every table contain per thousand parts: 40.5 calcium, 60.0 magnesium, 99.7 potassium,[2] 28.6 sodium, 60 manganese, 227 iron, 69 copper, 0.26 cobalt.

There is the lowly and often despised cabbage, now believed by experimenters to contain an element which will neutralize fall-out. It contains 0.38 phosphorus, 60.0 calcium, 60.0 magnesium, 99.7 of protective potassium, 8.6 sodium, 73 boron, 60 manganese, 277 iron, 69 copper, and 0.26 cobalt.

Lettuce, an everyday vegetable, contains at its latest analysis, 71.0 calcium, 49.3 manganese, 53.7 potassium, 12.2 sodium, 37 boron, 196 manganese, 227 iron, 60 copper, 0.19 cobalt.

All vegetables are not only food, but rich in various minerals and vitamins that are as medicine to the body.

Although herbs, roots, and barks have not as yet been fully analyzed, they are all rich in these elements, and it is possible that

1. Fifty years ago practically every mother knew how to roast or bake onions until soft, then squeeze out the juice and sweeten with honey to give to the children for colds, coughs, even croup or pneumonia. It has lost none of its virtues. The family physician was called only as a last resort.

2. It is now generally believed that lack of Potassium in the diet may be a cause of cancer, and that this mineral is required in the successful treatment of cancer.

these help in eliminating weaknesses since their medical properties remove congestions and eliminate disease.

These vegetables are all accepted as desirable. They are decidedly rich in medicinal elements and their value depends on the contents of the vitamin, mineral, and vital medicinal contents of these substances.

That universal delicacy, the mushroom, was considered a pure and simple fungus, also a poison. Now it is a great favorite with almost all people. Its richest element is iodine and, therefore, it is the ideal food for those suffering from under-development and goiter.

Seaweed, also known as Irish moss and by various other names, has the same value as the mushroom. It is rich in germ-plasm and iodine.

Next to be considered are a few of those plant products which still are classified as herbs. White oak bark was a universal favorite with the early Thomsonian and physiomedical physicians. Potash 70.00 parts per thousand of its mineral elements. Gout, rheumatism, intermittent fevers, chronic diarrhoea, and other sympathetic maladies continue to be treated with it.

Broom herb, the kidney remedy of the herbalists, contains 40.00 Potash in every 1,000 parts. Shave grass, the favorite kidney remedy of the German herbalists, is rich in calcium and silicon.

Who is there who does not like fruit and fruit drinks? Until lately, fruits helped to satisfy appetite, and fruit drinks were considered as soothing in fevers. Fruits also made appetizing wines. What are the real facts?

Wild cherry juice, whether fermented or unfermented, was always considered a tonic. The reason for this is its richness in iron oxide, potassium oxide and phosphoric acid.

Just as wild cherry was known as a tonic, so the juice of the black currant became known as an antiseptic, purifier of the blood, restorative of the nervous system, and an equally valuable remedy in anemia, malnutrition, and general debility. Why? Because it is rich in vitamins and positive alkali and contains, among other mineral elements, 13.70 potassium.

Who is not familiar with blackberry pie, blackberry wine and brandy, and the use of blackberry, especially dewberry-root tea for looseness of the bowels, particularly for children during the summer months? What are the facts? It contains per thousand parts: 19.68 potassium, 3.76 each of sodium and phosphorous, besides other valuable elements.

Consider the lowly parsley once used only to give an added taste to food. Now we know that it is rich in calcium, iron, thiamine, riboflavin, niacin and ascorbic acid. It is recognized by many physicians as valuable in the treatment of high blood pressure.

RENEWED INTEREST IN ONCE DISCARDED COMMON REMEDIES

It was not so long ago that the use of herbs as medicines was thought to be an old wives' tale. There has been a decided change in this concept and many physicians are replacing the chemical and synthetic preparations with them.

Roughly speaking, there are several reasons for the present rapidly increasing interest in herbal (organic) medicines: First may be the fact that it is becoming more and more difficult for the ill to obtain medical attention during the night, on Saturdays, Sundays, and holidays, even if living in towns or cities. Hence, a return to home (common) remedies.

Second, the fact that serious, highly legitimate newspapers are publishing lengthy articles on the revival of the interest of physicians in such remedies. In its October 28, 1959 edition, the Wall Street Journal published a lengthy article on the discovery that Snakeroot has great value in the treatment of high blood pressure, a condition that in one form or another is killing millions. Snakeroot is found in many states in America. Strangely enough, many whiskey drinkers placed the roots of this herb into their whiskey and drank it regularly. I noticed this habit with many men in my early years, and I know of none of them who died either from high blood pressure or heart disease.

Another lengthy article on the use of blueberry leaf tea or tincture in diabetes was published in the *National Weekly*, March 17, 1928.[3] Undoubtedly, hundreds of thousands of diabetics had recourse to this tea. Many continue to use it regularly. The physio-

---

3. Fully described in the chapter on household and domestic medicines and agents prescribed by liberal and natura physicians.

medicalist and Naturist prescribed the tincture (the fluid extract or tea made out of the leaves) in association with other natural remedies.

Vegetables are not merely vegetable nor are simply herbs or fruits simply fruits. They are what they are and serve their actual purpose, because of the organized mineral and vital (vitamin) elements they contain, and the various combinations of these elements as found in each separate specimen of plant life.

The Naturist or Natura physician studies each fruit and vegetable, familiarizes himself with its contents and then instructs the combining of two or more of them in order that the need may be supplied in each individual case. The Naturist is an investigator, an analyst, and a logician in arriving at his conclusions.

CONTENTS

1.

THE NATURA PHYSICIAN'S BASIS OF PROCEDURE

Disease (dis—ease, an un-ease) of whatever nature, is the result of some form of abnormal condition in a certain part, or parts of the body, brought about by a lack of certain elements necessary to proper physical functioning; procurable from the foods we consume and the liquids we drink, or as a result of congestion due to poor elimination.

It may logically be questioned: do not indiscretions frequently result in illness—an unnaturalness, unbalance, or lack of equilibrium? Assuredly so! However, the last phrase, *lack of* equilibrium is the answer.

Indiscretions or exposures use up, burn up, or consume. Life's activities are a process of consuming—burning up, combusting— certain elements in the body. If these elements are not immediately replaced, there will result an unbalance, which we term sickness, illness or disease. The reestablishment of balance demands immediate attention to supply the system with the elements lacking.

Under the natural plan or—if you will—the Divine Plan governing man, he continues strong, physically well, and virile by supplying his body with the elements being consumed, but only those required to maintain the balance, the equilibrium. All of these elements are obtainable from the organic (organized) kingdoms, principally the vegetables (this term including the herbs, roots and barks of certain trees). As indicated by Biblical inculcations or commands what are known as "herbs" are actually food that will supply the body with elements required to maintain a balance. Fruits, nuts, cereals, and even eggs, milk, and cheese come under this classification. The latter—milk, cheese, and eggs—are merely predigested and highly organized (vitalized) vegetables, grasses, and grains that have been consumed and converted—a form of predigestion—by the animal into proper food for man.

Certain plant life classified as herbals should no longer be known

1

as herbs, but as vegetables rich in food value as so long indicated by the Biblical statement in *Genesis,* a truth ignored because it was not generally understood.

Under natural law and the Divine order, non-organic (non-organized, i.e., synthetic) products of whatever nature, are abnormal and foreign to the human being (man as a body, mind, and Soul), and therefore detrimental. As man becomes conversant with natural laws and free from ignorance, he will be able to discard synthetics as food and medicine, because he will be conscious that the unnatural and unbalanced cannot bring about order and equilibrium in the highly organized economy of man.

Those who themselves follow this natural and sane law, as also those (physicians and teachers) who will help the weak and ignorant (the ill and discouraged), might well be classified as "vegetarians" though this term is too limited. Why not then call them naturists, since they follow the laws of Nature, harmonize their activities with them and refuse to accept the concepts of those who would set aside God's divine fiats by refusing to make use of the perfect, highly organized and correctly balanced element so freely placed before man for his use and welfare.

Under a new dispensation, wherein will function God's law, "medicine," as such: fruits, nuts, cereals, legumes, and vegetables, because of their contents will be so combined as to be both food and medicine, and among the now well known and frequently used vegetables will be included all the herbs. The Naturist will be both dietitian and herbalist, restricted by neither.

Experience taught early physicians the value of many plants.[4] Later the schools of practice commenced sending all plants to the chemical laboratory for experimentation, and when no active principle was found, discarded them.

The Naturist selects all of his plant life by their therapeutic properties and their organic mineral and vitamin content. These elements are assimilated by the human organism, carried throughout

---

4. This is not literally true. With few exceptions all the agents of which he made tinctures, fluid extracts, and powders had been used correctly and successfully by the crudely and unfairly dubbed "old wives" of Europe and the Indian women in America. All the physicians did was to refine them, establish accurate doses, and by experience find new uses for them. It is high time that we begin to give credit where credit is due.

the systems to the various cells, and by the law of selectivity chosen by these cells to be used for growth, for rebuilding themselves, and in maintaining or reestablishing health (equilibrium). The Natura physician does not attempt, or claim, to cure. He merely supplies the cells with the food (vegetables, herbs, cereals, legume, and fruits i.e., their vital mineral elements), which they need. By doing this he attempts to eradicate disease (cell weakness or cell congestion) and to establish a state of well-being. This has always been our plan of operation and the system we personally advocate.

Physical and Mental Reconstruction

The Natura physician does not profess to cure disease. In fact, no man, whatever his system, can do that. Nature *alone* is capable of curing (eliminating) disease, and she only can do so when the proper elements are supplied with which to rebuild the part of the body which has become weakened by disorganization.

All that we or any other man, however great he may be, can do is to seek the cause of the weakness, learn what the deficiencies are that brought it about, then proceed to supply the essential substances. Nature can then do the rebuilding—the reconstructing. There is no such thing as a physician as the word is commonly understood. The true physician is a teacher, one who includes the laws of life—a regimen of correct living, and who, if need be, supplies the substances required to eliminate the deficiencies of the ailing body.

The essential materials are *not* medicinal, but organic (organized) substances which we know as food (material ingested) that can be digested and assimilated by the hungry cells of the body. Drugs, those unorganized (nonorganized) substances so constantly pre-scribed, cannot be digested nor assimilated. They may be absorbed by the cells just as dyes are absorbed by cotton, woolen, or silk goods, but assimilation is not possible. As a result hungry cells are not supplied with the foods for which they are in crying need. Such agents are of no actual value, except in rare instances when they stimulate weakened (hungry and starved) cells to make greater effort to reestablish their lost balance.

The mistake of the modernists has been that they mistook absorption for assimilation. The human body is kept alive, normal, and active, only by the elements which the cells of the body can assimilate and build into themselves. Inorganic substances cannot be assimilated, although they may be absorbed.[5] Consequently, they do not become part of the cells, and give neither life nor strength to the cells. They may help in the elimination of congestions and in the reestablishment of equilibrium.

A Look into the Near Future

In the Natura, or newer science of medicine, when any abnormality (now known as a disease) manifests itself in an individual, the physical self will be examined carefully and scientifically and the lack—cause of the disease—discovered. The physician will then be able to know as a result of his diagnostic analysis, which of the many known elements are missing, and how to supply them.

The constituents (organic, mineral, and vitamin) of every vegetable including herbs, roots, and barks, and even the grasses are now well known, and the physician will prescribe them, either singly or in combination, in their natural state; and this will quickly and naturally tend to supply the need, the lack of which is the cause of the illness or lack of balance.

The coming enlightened practice, because of its naturalistic basis, will gradually replace all forms of serums and toxins now used in the field of therapeutics. Nature and Nature alone, will be the basis of all curative agents. This may appear to be a sweeping statement, but indications are already apparent that the change is taking place.[6]

---

5. Frequently, when this absorption does occur, the foreign substance remains in the system and forms a wedge between cells. This may be the beginning of tumors, cancers, and other abnormalities.

6. No criticism of any one prescribing serums, toxins, or synthetics is here intended. However, investigation quickly makes apparent that more and more people are accepting the Biblical concept that there shall be no blood pollution in any manner.

THE THOMSONIAN OR PHYSIO-MEDICAL
TREATMENT OF DISEASE

After long experience and a thorough investigation and examination of all the principal systems of medical practice, Prof. Curtis, a graduate of a regular school of Medicine, an able lecturer and founder of the first Physio-Medical College, said:

"There is a true science and practice called the 'Physio-Medical,' the character of which is indicated by its title. Its leaders are not men, but the immutable laws of Nature.

"It is not the gift or invention of any man or company, or succession of men. It is the eternal truth, science and art of God and his inestimable and unequalled gift to all who will receive and apply it properly.

"Different individuals in all ages and countries have discovered and promulgated more or less of its principles, and means and modes of practice, for which we should render to each one due honor and gratitude. And since, among them all, I know of no one who has given us so much that is true and good, connected with so little that is false and bad, as Dr. Samuel Thomson, so I know of no one who is entitled to higher honor or deeper and more lasting gratitude from all the sons and daughters of affliction than this man, of Alstead, New Hampshire, who presented to the world its chief medical discoveries and inventions in the ninth year of the last century.

"Other men may more clearly develop these God-given principles, remove from them errors and crudities that still cling to them, discover and devise better ways and means of applying them; but, I repeat, the doctrines themselves, the general deductions from them, and the character of the processes of medication which constitute the Physio-Medical science and practice, are the immutable truths and art devised by the unchangeable God for the benefit of the unchange-

5

able constitution of man, and can never 'progress' nor be supplanted while man shall inhabit this earth and disease continue to vex him.*

"This science and practice is the system of principles properly called physiological, or those that govern the formation and preservation of the organized body.

"(1) Its doctrines are that the human body is formed and controlled, preserved and defended, and, when injured, restored by the action of an invisible agent called the vital force; that, when all its parts are in such condition that this force can act freely and fully through them, this body is said to be in health.

"(2) The inability of any organ to perform its healthy function denotes disease. Hence, anything which in any way interferes with, or interrupts, this full, free and universal action through the body may be a cause of disease.

"(3) When, by ignorance, inadvertency, or unavoidable exposure, the conditions called disease have occurred, it teaches the duty of aiding the vital forces in its exciting, irritating and inflammatory efforts to remove the obstacles to healthy action, by means and process that do not further damage it, but tend directly to restore it [to supply requirements] and to heal the breach, if any.

"(4) It makes use of those articles and those only, which, in their nature, *harmonize with the organic tissues and the vital forces;* and, in the measure and mode of application required in any given case, directly aid that force in *restoring its equilibrium,* by judiciously removing or helping it to remove all the obstacles to its free and universal action.

"(5) It regards as poison anything and everything that is certainly known, in authorized medicinal doses or degrees, to have directly destroyed human life, or is, in its nature, calculated to deprive the organs of the power to respond to the action of the vital force in the production of irritation and fever, *viz.,* antimony, arsenic, mercury, belladonna, cantharides, cicuta, digitalis and other agents of like nature, and rejects these *in toto* from its remedial means.

---

* As long as man remains a physical creature, in part or whole, and as long as food is essential to his continuance, the Physio-Medical system of treatment is the natural and logical one, due to the fact that in each prescribed remedy there are elements required by the body of man just as there are in the food he daily consumes in order to rebuild the various parts of his body.

"(6) It adopts as remedial means and measures only those agents whose inherent tendency, like that of food, exercise, warmth, electricity and the influence of pleasant company, harmonize with the organic and conservative force of the system, and, like food and water, may and should be given or applied in the quantities and modes required, till the objects of their use are fully accomplished; till perfect health is established.

"There are three ways to aid man in the accomplishment of his object or wishes. The first is to remove the obstacles to his efforts; the second is to supply him with means best adapted to enable him to effect his purpose, and the third is to inspire him to exert all his own power and potencies in the right direction.

"In all cases of disease, there are, in the diseased parts, obstacles to the free and universal action of the nerves and circulating vessels, which the vital force is endeavoring to remove. The whole science of physiology consists in the knowledge of the character and uses of the organs and powers of the system; that of pathology so far as it is a science, in the knowledge of its conditions and wants; and the whole art of practice of medicine lies in the knowledge of the modes and the means of supplying the wants. In some cases, Nature requires but one, in others, two of the aids above indicated; in others, all. In some cases, all can be applied and supplied, by one means; in others, more are required.

"The Physio-Medical school commends the use of heat and moisture, bland diffusive stimulants, innocent astringents, of the character that may be taken in perfect health, in all the ways and to the extent ever required in disease, without seriously deranging the physiological state. Thousands of means and many processes are of this character, and may be used almost indifferently; but some of the best have been selected, as those that may be relied upon, since with them alone disease is treated and cured with as much directness and certainty as philosophical and chemical experiments are performed.

"Indeed, it can be easily proved that the best philosophers and chemists fail more frequently in the performance of their projected experiments, than do the well instructed and faithful Physio-Medical practitioners in the cure of disease.

"The conditions of their experiments being right, and the operators intelligent and skillful, both classes of operations are certain to produce the expected results. But sometimes the instrument or agent or both are defective, and then the results in neither case can succeed. The chemist can do nothing if his instruments are imperfect or his agents impure. So the physician can not cure a far gone case of tuberculosis with any medicine, nor any disease with inert substances.

"It is wonderful and a most astounding fact, that such a man as Samuel Thomson should have prescribed a hundred different remedies for the elimination of disease (many of which had never before been used), and yet among them all is not found a single deadly poison, nor even a dangerous substance.

"The simplicity of the Physio-Medical practice has been an objection to its universal application. It should be its greatest recommendation.

"The beauty and excellence of all science consists in its ability to reduce confusion to order, to extract philosophy from mystery, and to bring all the operations of art within the comprehension of the ordinary mind.

"The human body is supported and health sustained by the orderly process of digestion, circulation and disposition of a few organized substances, composed chiefly of carbon, oxygen hydrogen, nitrogen, phosphorus, lime and other organic mineral elements. All the motions of all the organs are produced by the simple contraction and relaxation of their constituent fibres.

"Disease is a condition that prevents this full, free, and regular action. All that is necessary to bring relief and establish order, is to remove obstacles to this action, and excite the organs to their proper motions. Whatever will invariably, promptly, powerfully and permanently relax, contract, and stimulate, will remove all obstructions to vital action, and cure all forms of disease, is a true medicine. As stimulation is nothing more than rapidly alternating relaxation and contraction [an interchange of activity as in the storage battery], it follows that the two motions in different ways and degrees of rapidity, sometimes relaxing, sometimes contracting, with greater or less velocity, are all that is necessary.

"We may discover new methods and means of carrying them out, and new modes of application, but the principles are the laws of man's nature and they cannot progress. Let these be adopted and consistently obeyed, and no longer is there any trouble about the 'secondary' action of the remedies for disease; no longer is the physician compelled to guess at the circumstances in which his remedies may be converted into poisons nor poisons into breast-milk; no longer to lift his club and strike, nor to raise his gun and fire at random, thus multiplying diseases and increasing their mortality. No longer must he grope without a clue, like Homer's Cyclops around his cave. But emancipated from the tyranny of the schools of physic and guided by the Physio-Medical principles, he sees at a glance, the character and conditions of disease; knows for a certainty the requirements and processes by which it may be routed, and proceeds to work in a scientific manner, with the same fixedness of principles and certainty of success that he would bring to bear upon the practice of any other art derived from the principles of its appropriate science. He cannot, indeed, expect to prolong human life forever, nor to reconstruct the organs of the body that may have been fatally marred; nor restore the functions of organs that are totally deprived of the power to perform them; but he can learn how to restore that which is capable of restoration, and he is blameworthy if he does anything to hasten dissolution, or entail upon his patient any chronic malady.

"It is impossible to perform a surgical operation of any magnitude without producing several injurious effects, each one of which argues against operations as a means of cure save in exceptional cases:

"1. The amount of vitality destroyed by the fear and dread of passing through an operation, combined with the operation frequently places cases beyond hope, a case that might easily have been cured if the correct treatment had been prescribed.

"2. To cut into the deep tissues of the body makes a severe wound in addition to the already existing condition. The amount of vitality required to heal such a wound draws heavily on the vital force of the patient.

"3. The anæsthetic usually administered under such circumstances still further reduces the vital force of the sufferer.

"4. The pain and weakness caused by the operation has a similar effect.

"Any one of these detrimental influences frequently is sufficient to bring about the death of a very weak patient.

"Consider for a moment the contrast: If, instead of fear, you substitute hope; if, in place of pain, you give ease and comfort; if, instead of benumbing and deadening the sensatory nerves with a poison, you stimulate and strengthen with a real medicine, the life of a patient is often saved when otherwise that life would be lost. It is an appalling fact that actual murder is often committed by performing needless surgical operations, and prescribing benumbing poisons as medicine.

"Why have old modes failed? Simply because the means employed were not adapted to accomplish the end desired.

"For instance, in speaking of a certain case, you will sometimes hear a physician say: 'I have tried everything, but nothing seems to do any good.' Now the real remedy or remedies suitable in the case he may be wholly ignorant of, consequently, he has not tried *everything*. The number of agents tried, even if millions, count for nothing, and most of them may actually have been harmful, if their tendency was not in line with the objective aimed at. A physician should be able to judge of this. Herein lies the test of his skill. The correct remedies have a tendency to produce the results sought, but a million non-indicated substances will have no power to bring relief and eradicate cause.

"One such authority, from whom we have quoted, made the claim that *all medicines are poisonous.* Now real medicines are not poisonous at all. One might just as well, and with equal truth, say that all foods are poisonous. The very nature of poison is to destroy living matter. True medicine is a substance which tends to supply necessary material to the bodily substances and to increase the life principle in man.

"Poisonous substances irritate and provoke the vital centers to increased activity, and frequently, *in spite* of being poisonous, if the person to whom given possesses a goodly degree of vitality, a cure will result. In such cases the drug, or drugs, act upon the inert system as does the driver's whip on the fagging horse. But poisons never add any permanent energy to the vital centers in man, and in cases where the force in these centers is very low, their effect is to exhaust it entirely and thus cause the death of the sufferer.

"Real medicine, whether in the form of an herb or a food, is a substance that will increase the energy in the vital centers without working any injury. Taking this view of the matter, a view which is the opinion of the foremost investigators at the present time and is substantiated by every experiment made by dietitians, it will be readily seen why the old school of medicine has been so frequently unsuccessful and has had to change from one theory to another, changing from poisons to toxins and serums of animal origin, and why they have been disappointed in the results obtained."

It will also be recognized by every thinking man, that if we are to gain our object, we must take the right course, employing the means and measures necessary to success. There are hundreds of non-poisonous remedies now in use which are being more and more substituted for the poisonous drugs formerly prescribed and to the great benefit of all concerned.

Every one, whether physician or layman, who holds in his hands the life of a human being, should seriously consider what an awful thing it is to give a drug the *tendency* of which is to *destroy,* while trying to cure. To say the least, it is an exceedingly contradictory, and unreasonable act.

This is another confession made by some of the most eminent physicians in their ignorance of the real nature of physiological disorders called disease, and the uncertainty of the action of their remedies; hence, their conclusion, "medicine is not a science." It is not to be wondered at, that they came to this conclusion, when we take even a cursory glance at the unscientific remedial agents and methods which they employ in their efforts to cure. There has been too much false reasoning in regard to medicine. For instance, a physician or patient complains that a certain remedy has lost its effect. If we use reason and consider for a moment, we will quickly see that the nature of a remedy, in itself, never changes. This is a fact of the greatest importance. On this point, Prof. Kirk of Edinburgh, Scotland, says:

" 'Circumstances change but essential natures never. A remedy is always the same in nature, and will have the same effect whenever it is used in the same circumstances. It is not wise, merely to say that the remedy has lost its effect and throw it aside as useless. True skill in such a case looks to the circumstances. The remedy has done all it could reasonably be expected to do; but the circumstances have changed, and another effect is now required.

" 'When we take the common sense view of the matter we are left free to discover the real remedy. We have seen the benefit of this many times over when the actual remedy was found, applied, and the patient cured. This remedy has often proved in many cases exceedingly simple. For instance, we have placed a finger on the root of a nerve supplying the muscles to the part in which the pain was felt and that pain instantly ceased. We have continued the treatment for perhaps half an hour or so and the pain did not return. We were told that all our remedies had failed. Every one of those remedies had had its true effect and had never lost that, only it was another remedy that was required. What was needed was only a little knowledge of the wondrous system of the living frame of man. It is a most precious gift that is given to all who accept it, that of knowing how to pass from a remedy when it is not the right one, and so be open to find the correct one. Let us gain a real understanding of the nature of all things with which we have to deal, and let us work on that understanding. God himself [the functioning Law] will teach us when we are willing to follow in the light offered us.' "

3.

BASIC PRINCIPLES OF THE NATURA SYSTEM

1. *Matter,* in all its diversity of character, quality, form and combination, may be classified into two great divisions, namely: *Organic* and *inorganic.*

2. *Organic* matter includes the two vast kingdoms of Nature: the *animal* (brute and man) and the *vegetable.*

3. *Inorganic* matter includes all bodies not possessed of *conscious* life, or such as are not endowed with a capacity for life, that is, *free movement.*

4. *Inorganic* and *dead* matter is controlled or governed by laws of force, embracing chemistry and physics and natural philosophy.

5. *Organic* or *living* bodies, though influenced to a certain extent by the laws which govern inorganic matter, are sustained in their living state by *vital* laws. These laws hold supremacy over and control those of physics and chemistry, which they modify and render subservient on many occasions to the purpose of vitality.

6. The principle of life is the same in all animated beings; and the human animal economy is governed by the same general laws as that of the truly human economy.

7. *Life,* or the *living* state, is a series of actions and reactions, or motions in animal matter, of which organized bodies are alone susceptible, and it may be truthfully said of them that "activity is life."

8. Without *organization* there cannot be life. Again, organized bodies, though possessed of a *capacity for life,* require the aid of stimulants (active agents) to call them into activity.

9. Animal life can be supported only by external means obtained by it or supplied to it.

10. *Life* is created and kept functioning by the influence of *heat* or *caloric* activity upon *organized* bodies.

11. *Heat,* or *caloric activity,* is the *power* or *agency* by which other stimulants such as atmospheric air, light, electricity, galvanism, food, drink, medicine, and all *reconstructing* agents are made to act upon the system.

12. *Caloric activity* brings into play that power (an electro-galvanic potency, since life is the result of action and reaction, negative upon positive, acid upon alkali) which is the immediate agent of those varied and complicated actions which form and fashion the organs; conveys to and appropriates nourishment to every organ and tissue; *sustains animal matter in a state of composition;* selects and expels effete or worn out matter by the pores of the skin, the kidneys, and other depuratory organs; carries on all the various secretions and enables the organs to react against or resist the influences that tend to their destruction.

These last two propositions form the cornerstone, or basis, of the physio-medical art of medicine.[1]

13. In the early period of animal life (during the embryonic stage) until the organs become developed, heat is derived from the mother. As the organs become developed, they are endowed with the power of producing or generating heat. After birth the supply of animal heat is dependent upon this function of calorification, or heat generating power; thus *vital* action, first produced by heat, creates the power, or generates the influence necessary to the continuance of its action. Heat is evolved in every part of the system, and the amount of caloric activity generated will be proportionate as the vital action is greater.

14. As the heat of the system is lessened, vital action will diminish in that proportion. If the system is deprived of caloric activity for a certain length of time, all the preservative, recuperative, and sanative phenomena cease. It is the same with oxygen.

15. The stomach is the seat or "throne" of the vital powers; the main center, or source, with heat and oxygen carries on and governs the important vital functions of circulation, respiration, digestion, nutrition, assimilation, and the activity of the various secretions.

---

1. Presently the Natura system.

16. The stomach is in almost every instance the seat of disease. When this organ is disordered,[2] the power of generating heat and nervous energy is diminished, and consequently the actions and functions of other organs, especially that of the liver, become weakened or deranged. In fever (temperature due to the extra efforts of the vital organs to throw out the enemies of life), although the heat of the surface is increased above the natural standard, the amount of heat generated may be less than is produced in a state of health. The secretions and transpirations from the skin and mucous surface being suspended, the heat is locked up in the system. This, contrary to popular belief, is a wise provision for retaining the heat, in order to sustain the recuperative actions, and thus effect a crisis in disease. Experiments have shown that in most inflammatory diseases, the blood contains less positive electricity than it does when taken from one in health. As the functions of the stomach and bowels are restored to a healthy condition, a natural warmth and activity become established throughout the system.

17. The same means that will restore the natural temperature of the system, as do pure stimulants (*Capsicum,* for instance) and the vapor baths, will also increase the electrogalvanic, or nervous power, which governs the circulation and all the vital functions. It is to be noted *especially* that the healthy activity of the digestive powers is due to the saliva—*alkaline*—mixed with the food we eat and which comes in contact with the digestive *acids* in the stomach. There is an electrogalvanic activity set in motion just as we find it in the modern storage battery.

18. As the natural warmth of the system is reduced, either from a disordered stomach or from any other cause, the nervous power which maintains an equilibrium (equilibrium alone is health) in the circulation is enfeebled; hence in disease a loss of the natural balance of equilibrium in the circulation of the blood is a common occurrence.

19. An undue accumulation of blood in any part of the body is attended by a deficiency (unbalance) in other parts. Thus in fevers there is an unnatural quantity of blood at the surface, and a corresponding lack inwardly; determinations of blood to the head are accompanied with a loss in the lower extremities.

---

2. The importance of a proper diet which sustains, and supports but does not congest, is here indicated.

20. The same means that will correct a disordered stomach and "raise the heat" of the system to its natural standard will tend to restore the natural balance to the circulation of the blood.

21. As the natural heat and nervous power are reduced, either by a cold (congestion interfering with proper circulation), disordered stomach (interference with the interblending of acids and alkalies), or by any other cause whatsoever, the functioning of digestion, nutrition, and assimilation becomes enfeebled or disordered. The same cause also deranges the secreting organs, as the liver and glands of the mucous membranes. In many instances in disease, the liver (the most important organ in the body of man) ceases to secrete bile; and the excessive thirst accompanying fever arises from diminished or suspended secretions of the glands of the mucous membrane.

Relative to this last proposition, it may be said in passing that if the activity of the liver could be maintained at normal, man would never know disease, would not grow old, would always be happy, never know a "blue" moment, and quickly elevate himself to the plane of the "gods."

22. Whatever will cleanse the stomach, restore the natural heat, and produce perspiration will also tend to restore the digestion, assimilation, secretions, and in fine remove every derangement which occurs in disease.

23. The lower order of animals, as in the hibernating species, can bear the abstraction of heat from their bodies without producing disorganization; they sink into a state of torpor and insensibility during winter, and on the return of warm weather are reawakened into life and activity.

24. In the higher order of animals, and in man, the abstraction of heat can be borne below a certain degree only for a limited period without producing disorganization and death. Hence, they are endowed with a power to *react* against cold and other deleterious agents; and by thus establishing a counteracting force or influence, life and organization are preserved against causes tending to their destruction. Many of the symptoms which occur in disease, such as pain and a state of fever, are caused by the recuperative, life-sustaining activity, the organs being driven, as it were, to a new mode of

action with the design of counteracting the influence of offending causes and regaining their lost vitality.

25. *Fever* (rise or fall in temperature) does *not* constitute a disease but is *always an evidence* of the existence of an *offending cause* in the system, a friendly warning that nature is struggling to remove such a cause.

26. Living creatures are ever surrounded by agents or forces which exert an influence in direct antagonism to the laws of life and tend to subvert or destroy vital action. Thus the living state is held, as it were, in a balance between opposing powers.

27. The direct effect of cold and other morbific agents upon the system is to weaken vital action and to lessen the power of generating heat: hence, disease of every form and variety commences with symptoms which show that the vital powers are weakened; these are *lassitude, general debility, coldness of the surface and extremities, and chilliness.* Cold and damp feet exert an influence in weakening and deranging the natural and healthy order of activity in the system, and thus prove a fruitful source of disease, yet would be powerless if there were no congestions present in the system due to an improper diet, inactivity, and various other causes. Dampness operates as a conducting medium by which the caloric activity, and more especially the electrogalvanic fluids, escape not only from the lower extremities, but also from the digestive functions and all the viscera of the abdomen by means of the nerves, which form a connecting chain of conductors or channels throughout the system for the passage or circulation of this nerve fluid. As the nervous influence escapes from the system, the functions, over which it has control, become enfeebled and deranged.

28. The first symptoms in disease prove a weakened condition of vital activity. As the constitution reacts, a new train of symptoms ensues. The pulse becomes quicker and stronger, the surface becomes hot and dry, and the system is in a state of feverish excitement; in other words, the patient has a fever—the battle between the destructive and constructive agents is on. The constitution with all its constructive agents struggles against disease and occasions the fever, and it is by this power of reaction that disease is overcome.

Intermittent fever, as it is termed, commences with a chill. As the system reacts, fever ensues; and the recuperative efforts which occasion the temperature, restore the heat, bringing on perspiration and frequently other critical evacuations, more especially from the kidneys, by which the disease is partly or wholly removed until the return of the succeeding chill when the constitution institutes the same preservative, recuperative activity. In the *eruptive* diseases which are always of zymotic (inner filth) origin, as smallpox, measles, chickenpox, and scarlet fever there is always in the commencement a general debility, chilliness, and a disordered stomach. These are the direct effects of the morbific agents that produce the disease; and but for a counteracting influence, vital action would be quickly overcome. The constitution (stored vital force) establishes a reaction or fever, by which the disease is thrown to the surface, producing an eruption on the skin.

29. The design of reaction or fever is to restore the lost heat and vitality, *and to remove all morbific or deleterious agents and their effects from the system,* and thus preserve it from destruction.

30. A course of treatment that will cleanse the stomach and bowels and restore their natural activity and at the same time remove obstructions from the system will automatically eliminate fever, by assisting to bring about what the fever is endeavoring to accomplish. When the offending cause is removed, there will be nothing to excite fever or reaction.

There is another and directly opposite plan (that at present almost universally practiced) for subduing fever, to wit: Reduce the vital forces or the recuperative efforts of nature. This, though the fashionable and accepted practice, is nevertheless directly against nature's laws, is frequently unsuccessful, and is hazardous to future health, if not to the life, of the patients on whom it is tried.

There is hardly a person who has never had nothing more than the la grippe or influenza, who is not suffering from some weakness. This is absolutely nothing less than the aftereffects of the fashionable treatment frequently prescribed.

31. One of the most important indications in the treatment of all acute diseases attended with high arterial excitement or violent fever, is to overcome the contracted or spasmodic condition of the capillary vessels by relaxing the system and cleansing the stomach with the one universal and non-harmful agent—*Lobelia.*

32. To effect such a relaxation of the system there is probably no agent of equal value. This medicine exerts a surprising influence in equalizing the nervous power and in relaxing the system *without* in any way weakening the vital properties. In many instances, however, fever and its cause may be removed by the same means that alone will overcome a chill, i.e., pure stimulants and vapor or hot baths, vapor baths preferred. According to the physio-medical philosophy, medical men of the dominant school have not made a proper distinction between true stimulants that strengthen and promote a healthy action and those agents which occasion morbid excitement, at the expense of the vital forces. Brandy and other alcoholics, frequently excellent medicines at the very onset of a cold, generally aggravate fevers, and hence it has been inferred that all stimulants are improper in such cases. A patient who would be injured by brandy would be benefitted, in the same condition, by taking one grain of *Capsicum* every 30 minutes.

33. As a consequence of a reduction and derangement of vital action, there are, in disease, thickened, morbid secretions, termed "canker" by Dr. Thomson. These are formed on the lining membrane of the stomach and bowels and indicated by "cold sores" in the mouth. In acute diseases, as in dysentery, pleurisy, various forms of eruptive diseases, and all other febrile affections, there is a tendency more or less, to putrefaction, which proves deleterious to the constitution. The stomach becoming coated with thickened, tenacious secretions or "canker," is a general cause of a disease being protracted as this indicates a "low" state.

It was an observation of Dr. Thomson, that "where there is a settled fever there is canker seated in the stomach." The tongue, as stated, is more or less coated with cankerous or morbid secretions, and its appearance affords a criterion by which to judge the condition of the entire mucous membrane. The tendency to soften and clean off this canker from the edges of the tongue is usually one of the first and most favorable signs of the successful passing of a crisis.

34. To free the mucous membranes from canker is the primary importance in the cure of disease. This requires, in the first place, the use of agents that will excite the secretions and restore the inward or natural heat by which, as Dr. Thomson expressed it, "the canker is

brought to a point," and as these morbid secretions soften they may be removed.

First of all then, the stomach should be cleansed thoroughly by the reasonable use of *Lobelia* and warm water. After the stomach is freed of its foul contents, always present in fevers of every description, the vital forces are reinforced with *capsicum* and the morbid condition of the entire system is protected by *Echinacea*. Here we have three sovereign remedies, and all of vegetable origin. In fact, these are not medicines, but true foods supplying the system with material that it requires to balance itself.

35. In violent local determination of blood to a part or organ, as in croup, inflammation of the brain, violent pleurisy, inflammation of the kidneys, apoplexy, and other like diseases, one of the most important indications in the treatment is to overcome this undue determination of the blood to the affected part by relaxing the system with Indian tobacco, either *via* the stomach or administered by means of the internal bath.

36. Finally, we believe that the physiomedical system[3] fulfills all the important requirements for the treatment of the ailing; and when scientifically applied (with reason and understanding), it will bring about a balance and equilibrium, which is, generally speaking, a cure.

---

3. The present Natura system which includes the Thomsonian and physiomedical.

4.

EMETICS IN THE ELIMINATION OF DISEASE

In the Thomsonian system of practice, emetics constituted the most effectual agency employed in the treatment of disease (the relief of indispositions). There is scarcely a form of sickness in which the use of emetics as a prompt cleansing agent will not prove beneficial, and in many instances they are indispensibly necessary to the recovery of the patient.[1] Previous to the discoverey of the medical properties of Indian tobacco by Samuel Thomson, poisonous substances were employed almost exclusively as emetics.

In many cases of slight or sudden attacks of disease, all that is required by the operation of an emetic is to throw off the foul contents of the stomach which had oppressed and deranged its functions. But where disease has become chronic, other important remedial agents are essential. They relax the system, and in this way overcome obstructions, equalize the circulation of the blood and the nervous influence—invigorate the energies of the stomach, and remove morbid secretions from its mucous surface; restore the secretions, and in fact, assist the constitution in resisting disease, and thus aid her efforts in reestablishing a state of health.

If there is a general fever pervading the body, it is evidence of an abnormal condition of the stomach; and hence at the very onset of fever, the use of emetics is particularly indicated. Whenever a fever arises from the cause of undigested food, worms in the intestines, the stomach's energies sunken or its functions prostrated by poisonous influences or previous exposure to cold, emetics are indicated.

In measles, scarlet fever, and smallpox the disease will be rendered more mild in character, less dangerous, and frequently of

---

1. From mother nature learn wisdom is one of God's greatest commands. For instance, watch the action of a sick animal, especially the dog. First of all, it refuses all food; next it will eat grasses or herbs until it is able to empty its stomach, then it rests until the normal functioning of the organ is established, when it will again accept food. Animals who follow this plan seldom die of disease.

21

shorter duration by the early administration of emetics to thoroughly cleanse the stomach.

In the disease of children, emetics constitute by far the most efficient remedy. Vomiting is nature's method of relieving the stomach in infancy. The vomiting of a child after feeding is the most certain indication that its digestive organism is functioning properly. We can not do wrong in giving emetics to sick children, more especially at an early stage of disease. In sudden attacks of fever, croup, convulsions, or in cases of acute indigestion (so-called heart failure), *Lobelia* should be given, either in powder in warm teas, in tablet form with warm water, the tincture in warm water, or the third preparation of Thomson. The latter is particularly adapted to cases of spasms and when the heat of the system is very low, as also in advanced stages of disease. No danger need be apprehended from vomiting a child too much in croup, nor in any other form of violent attacks of disease.

In protracted chills, where the patient is in a stupor, the third preparation of *Lobelia* should be freely given, with the application of external warmth and friction to the surface with a view of bringing on a reaction. When there is unconsciousness, any preparation of *Lobelia* may be freely given *via* the bowels by the use of the internal bath or Murphy drip.

Emetics administered in the early period of scarlet fever will frequently exert a powerful influence in moderating the violence and in shortening the duration of this dreaded disease.

In bleeding from the lungs, the effect of the operation is to attract blood from the lungs and diffuse it through the system, by which the bleeding will be checked. Warm foot baths, or the vapor bath, should be employed to aid in restoring the natural equilibrium of the circulation of the blood.

In bleeding from the stomach, in which blood will be raised by vomiting, the employment of active emetics are indicated, not only to dislodge accumulations of blood in the stomach, which may have oppressed its energies, but to cause a distribution of the blood throughout the system and to strengthen the weakened capillary vessels of the mucous membrane of the stomach. The third preparation of *Lobelia* given freely, together with the application of the vapor bath when possible, is generally successful in the treatment of bleeding from the stomach, and it is not known ever to have failed in checking the hemorrhage.

In uterine hemorrhage the flow of blood frequently may be controlled by active emetics, aided by the injection of geranium and bayberry directly to the parts, or packing with cotton which has been saturated with this combination.

In severe colds and sore throat, either from inflammation or the existence of ulcers, emetics are of great benefit.

Emetics are more effectual than any other remedy in the relief of bronchitis and other forms of disease of the chest. The most severe paroxysms of asthma may be overcome by a thorough emetic, more especially when the emetic is preceded by the application of a vapor bath, rendering the system more sensitive to the impression of medicine.

In pleurisy and inflammation of the lungs, emetics may be employed with great advantage, especially in the early period of the disease. The act of vomiting is not attended with any great pain or difficulty in the most violent attacks of pleurisy or inflammation of the lungs. As the patient becomes nauseated from the action of the emetic, the system is relaxed, which is the explanation why a patient may vomit with so little pain or difficulty in active inflammation in the pleura or lungs.

In their wide and pervading operation emetics subdue, or have a tendency to subdue, vascular activtity to remove cutaneous constriction, promote absorption from the lungs, facilitate expectoration, lessen dyspnœa cough, and sanguinous discharge, also calm the system by equalizing excitement, and thus reestablishing that just balance in the distribution of the blood, on which the restoration and maintenance of health so materially depends.

In whooping cough more benefit may be derived from the use of emetics than from any other single remedy. In violent cases an emetic should be given daily, or even two or three times a day. In those cases when violent paroxysms of coughing are observed to come on at certain periods, it is a good practice to place the patient under the influence of *Lobelia,* even giving the amount necessary to induce vomiting previous to the time at which the paroxysms of coughing usually occur.

Emetics form an important part of the treatment for rheumatism, lumbago, gout, neuralgia, etc. No remedy under my observation produces so much relief in these forms of disease as an active emetic, and the efficiency is greatly enhanced by the previous application of a vapor bath. The reason why these emetics are of so great a value is due to their power to establish a balance in the system—an equilibrium.

Of the various remedies that have been employed in the treatment of dyspepsia emetics have proved the most successful. Even in those cases where there is extreme tenderness at the pit of the stomach, an emetic after a vapor bath will afford more and quicker relief in general than any other remedy. In the early stage of dyspepsia, digestion in most instances may be restored by one or two active emetics followed by the free use of *Capsicum* with the meals.

Sick-headache, depending upon a disordered condition of the stomach, may be speedily relieved by an emetic.

Emetics are well adapted in the relief of every variety of colic or cramp of the stomach. In diarrhoea, dysentery, and cholera morbus, digestion is *nil,* and the stomach contains more or less foul matter, and its mucous surface is coated with thickened secretions interfering with its functions, which naturally increases the distress of the latter and favors the disease. To excite free vomiting is particularly indicated in the treatment of such disorders. Besides relieving the stomach of foul matter and giving tone to the organ, such emetics exert a beneficial influence upon the secretions, causing a determination of the blood to the surface, restoring capillary circulation, and aiding the efforts of nature to restore healthy activity in the mucous membrane of the bowels.

Epilepsy, or falling sickness as it is most generally known, is in many instances traceable to a congested or otherwise disordered condition of the stomach and indicates the employment of emetics. By exhibiting them just *before* the time for the onset of a paroxysm, they will frequently prevent it, and even if they fail wholly to do this they render the spasms milder and of shorter duration. Nor is this all they accomplish; for by the strong and direct impression made on the stomach and nervous system, the commencement in that organ of the wrong association constituting the disease is broken, and it will yield more readily to indicated remedies.

Nearly the same view may be taken of hysteria. Even admitting that the disease is mostly the result of a congested uterus, it frequently does proceed from gastric irritation and demands to be treated accordingly. Whatever may be the immediate cause of the paroxysm, no remedy is so quickly effective as an emetic. It promptly allays the convulsive agitation of the nervous system and creates a state of mental composure that invites restorative sleep.

The best plan is always to give an emetic during the paroxysm to shorten its duration, and afterwards treat the cause which will usually be found to have its seat in the uterus. It may be an irritated or ulcerated womb, which directly affects the nervous system and brings about the paroxysm. *Lobelia* is of *immense* value in preventing the tension of the nervous system. The uterus, in the meantime, must be treated for the cause. When that is removed, the effect will cease.

Apoplexy, brought on as it so frequently is by a mass of undigested food in the stomach, calls for a free exhibition of emetics, of which the third preparation of *Lobelia* is appropriate. It should also be administered by enema and allowed to be retained in the bowels to assist in exciting vomiting, to relax the system, and equalize the nervous system. Even if the seat of apoplexy should be in the brain, and considered incurable, the treatment indicated will be of benefit, and it is always harmless. Many forms of mania or neurotic symptoms are frequently the result of a disordered condition of the stomach, and many cases have been permanently cured by first freely prescribing emetics and then restoring the tone and functions of the digestive organism.

In chronic dyspepsia, as in other forms of deeply-seated diseases, the mucous membrance of the stomach becomes more or less coated with a false and morbid membrane; a general torpor then pervades the system, the nervous energy is protracted, and the activity of the mind is greatly depressed. In such cases there is no plan of treatment that offers equal success comparable with that of the frequent use of the pack bath and stimulating emetics. This plan will prove the most effectual in restoring the secretions and bringing about the detachment and removal of false membranes lining the stomach. Without effecting this in some manner, the functions of the stomach cannot be permanently restored. It has been observed, and this should be borne in mind, that patients who have long been affected with dyspepsia are very liable to experience severe pains under the operation of an emetic and complain of feeling worse about the time the disease is taking a *favorable* turn.

Affections of the head, in general, proceed from derangement of the stomach; so that not only in sick-headache are emetics indicated, but also the most violent neuralgic pains in the head, accompanied with extreme tenderness of the scalp, will be relieved promptly by an emetic which acts freely in emptying the stomach. Even genuine *tic-douloureux,* the neuralgia of the face, has been overcome by the same practice, and with such facility as to place it decidedly above all other modes of treating this most painful, and hitherto nearly unmanageable, affection.

The operation of emetics in conjunction with the vapor or pack baths are applicable to cases of dropsy. Besides cleansing the stomach and placing the system under the relaxing influence of *Lobelia,* they promote the action of the absorbent vessels, and consequently the use of the remedy is particularly well adapted to such conditions.

Emetics form an important part of the treatment in the cure of jaundice as it is of the utmost importance to free the stomach of all morbid matter, thoroughily cleansing and toning it. Many cases of this disease are quickly cured by the administration of *Lobelia* and followed by stimulating compositions. Cases that are deeply seated will require, as do other forms of settled (chronic) disease, a repetition of the course of medicine together with the indicated intermediate treatment.

Torpor of the liver, which attends jaundice and bilious fever, is generally removed, and the functions of this important organ restored through the influence of vapor or pack baths and active emetics. To restore the natural temperature of the body, impart electricity, relax the system with *Lobelia;* and together with the influence of straining efforts to free the stomach of congestice matter, this constitutes the most effectual means of relieving congestion of the liver and of quickly restoring its functions. *Lobelia* administered *via* enema and retained exerts the same beneficial influence upon the system as when administered *via* the stomach, and if for any reason the stomach will not retain a medicine this is the proper way to administer it. Many sufferers will not permit any medicine to be given to them to cause vomiting, as they labor under the mistaken impression that such a medicine is not indicated in *their* case. The physician will, therefore, be wise when dealing with this class of patients and administer *Lobelia* by means of the internal *bath,* the enema.

Whenever the system experiences a severe shock, as by falling from a height, a violent blow, or by a severe burn or scald, digestion will be suspended; and if the accident should occur soon after, or even within an hour or two after the patient has partaken of a heavy meal, the stomach should immediately be evacuated by an active emetic. This may save the patient a great deal of suffering and will materially lessen the danger of the injury.

Emetics like *Lobelia* may be employed with perfect safety during every stage of pregnancy. Most of the derangements of the system consequent upon that state, such as a feeling of fullness, dizziness, or violent pain in the head, pain and distress in the back and loins, extreme sickness, water brash—*that most disagreeable affliction*—and distress at the stomach, may be quickly relieved and entirely eliminated by the active Lobelia emetic preceded by the use of an enema and the sheet ablution. Women carried through several complete courses of medicine during the two weeks preceding their confinement, *invariably* derive great benefit and complete relief from distress by this method. A full course of medicine administered just before confinement is incomparably the best plan that has ever been adopted for insuring an easy and safe labor.

Puerperal fever, convulsions, and other forms of disease which sometimes are resultant on confinement may, in the greater number of instances, be prevented or at least the system be placed in a far better condition to resist the influence of the exciting cause of the disease by a course of medicine.

The condition of the stomach always excites a controlling influence over local diseases, such as painful swellings in every part of the body, swollen breasts, swellings in the groin, neuralgia, local inflammations, gout, diseases of the kidneys, carbuncles, affections of the spine, and abscesses. In the early stage painful swellings can be brought to a crisis and dispersed without suppuration taking place by giving vapor or pack baths and emetics, together with a proper use of the enema to assist the action of the bowels in cleansing the system of impurities.

Just in the proportion as the stomach is disordered, will local diseases become more difficult to cure. On the contrary, indolent ulcers of several years standing have been healed in a few weeks, chiefly by improving the condition of the system generally and more particularly that of the stomach by courses of medicine of which the emetic constituted the most important part of the treatment; elimination of morbid matter being the first requisite in the cure of disease irrespective of its nature or location.

Even when the seat of disease is located principally in the brain, emetics may be given with great advantage. This is because the brain is actually the positive section (station) of the nervous system—the solar plexus being the other—the negative. Whatever affects the nervous system, even in a small way, will most certainly and directly affect the brain. *Lobelia* has its greatest influence on the nervous system, and consequently its effects on the brain are just as great as on any part of the nervous system.

The stomach possesses a very low degree of sensibility so that its functions may be greatly depleted or disordered without the patient experiencing any symptoms of disease, except in parts remote from the stomach. One who is subject to a weakness in any part of the spine will experience an increase of the trouble when the stomach becomes more disordered than usual. In many instances disease of the spine has been eliminated by the use of pack baths and emetics.

Eruptions of the skin, such as scald head, nettlerash, and eczema, are frequently occasioned by derangement of the digestive functions, and these eruptions may be effectually treated by emetics followed by proper medication.

Only a sufficient amount of Lobelia should be given to cause the sufferer to vomit freely; immediately thereafter tonics prescribed to give heat and strength to the patient.

Lastly every man, woman, and child would benefit beyond expectation by fortnightly cleansing the stomach by the use of *Lobelia,* and this followed by a stomach bitters.

5.

STEAM, OR VAPOR, AND PACK BATHS

Although the use of the vapor or steam bath as a means of curing disease was employed many centuries ago, the principle upon which it operates in removing disease was not fully explained, nor its utility in aiding the operation of medicine recognized or appreciated, until Dr. Thomson began to utilize it in the elimination of those factors which cause disease in the human system.

The vapor or steam bath constitutes an important part of the Thomsonian system of practice fulfilling several important indications in the relief of the ailing. It diffuses warmth through the system, equalizes the circulation, imparts electricity to the blood, and increases the sensibilities of the system to the impressions of medicine.

"In all cases," said Dr. Thomson, "where the heat of the body is so far exhausted as not to be rekindled by using the medicines, and being shielded from the surrounding air by a blanket, or being in bed, and chills or stupor attend the patient, then applied heat by steaming becomes indispensable. Heat caused by steam in the manner I use it is more natural in producing perspiration than any dry heat that can be applied to the body in any other manner, for a dry heat will only serve to dry the air and prevent perspiration in many cases of disease, where a steam by water, or vinegar and water, will promote perspiration and add a natural warmth to the body, thereby increasing the power of life and motion and aid greatly in removing disease."

There is scarcely a form of disease or a condition of the system in which the steam bath may not be employed not only with safety but with decided benefit. One of the most important results of the application of the bath is adding warmth to and invigorating the blood. It has been ascertained that in disease even of the most inflammatory character, the blood contains less electricity than it does when in a healthy condition, and by the employment of these baths in the early stages of many diseases, they may be quickly removed.

To diseases of an inflammatory character preceded by colds, with exception of erysipelas, vapor or steam bath bring quick relief.

These baths may also be employed with immense benefit in diseases of the urinary organs (strangury, gravel, and retention of urine) and inflammation of the lungs.

Slight attacks of jaundice can be relieved in many instances by a single vapor bath, followed by an emetic and then a stimulant. In croup, where the disease has continued several hours, the vapor bath (vinegar added to the water) is almost indispensable in order to restore the natural warmth of the blood and assist the operation of medicine.

In asthma when the system is in a cold and torpid condition, medicine will frequently fail to afford much relief. In this form of disease, it has been found that the hot air bath is as effectual as the vapor bath, and this may be administered with much less trouble.

In eruptive diseases, such as smallpox, scarlet fever, varioloid, and measles, the vapor bath may be used with benefit at any stage of the disease though, in these cases, the pack bath is to be preferred. If the eruption is slow to appear, applying a vapor bath will bring it to the surface. Or if there is a tendency to retrocession of the eruption, the vapor bath should be applied, or at least a moist heat applied, around the patient; and a powerful stimulant administered, such as the third preparation of *Lobelia;* and a stimulating injection given. In every stage of smallpox, the vapor bath is grateful to the patient and aids the constitution in throwing out the disease. In the later period of eruptive diseases, when scabs are forming and the patient is much distressed, the steam bath will afford more relief than any other means that can be employed, and when the scales are dry and falling off there is no better remedy for restoring the natural healthy condition of the skin. Scarlet fever and measles are very liable to be followed by dropsy, running of ears, swelling of glands, etc. arising in part from an unhealthy condition of the skin, which may be remedied by steam baths.

In violent colds and catarrh where the breathing is greatly oppressed and the skin dry and drawn, or cold and clammy, and the patient is much distressed, the employment of vapor baths becomes highly beneficial not only to relieve the distressing symptoms but to facilitate to operation of medicine.

In peritonitis, which is a most fatal form of disease after it has progressed to a certain stage, the vapor bath should be promptly and perseveringly applied, besides giving *Lobelia* to relax the system and such remedies as *Echinacea* and *Myrrh* to overcome the morbidity.

In inflammation of the lungs, liver, stomach, and bowels, or any other of the internal organs, the vapor bath will be found to relieve pain, assist the operation of medicine, and shorten the course of the disease.

In "low fevers," as they are termed by the laity, where the heat and vitality of the sufferer are far reduced there is a marked benefit from the use of these baths. A patient too weak to sit up or even raise his head will bear steaming on a couch or mattress, provided provided proper attention be given to bathe the face and surface of the body occasionally with alcohol.

These baths form an important auxiliary in the treatment of rheumatism, gout, lumbago, palsy, hysteria, chlorosis, neuralgia, consumption, all fevers, scrofula, etc. Finally, the application of warmth to the body by means of steam aids the efforts of nature to overcome every kind of disease that is curable.

The steam bath affords a protection to the system against the invasion of disease, and when applied in the early stage of many forms of disease will effectually prevent it becoming settled, by restoring the lost heat, promoting the secretions, and removing obstructions.

If the efficacy and safety of the steam bath in midwifery were generally known, the practice of giving ergot and other agents of like nature, would eventually be substituted. By means of the vapor bath and *Lobelia,* the muscles may be more effectually relaxed than by any others means and at the same time the secretions are promoted and nature assisted without the least possible degree of danger to the patient. For pain in the back and loins during pregnancy, the steam bath may be used with great benefit.

As a course of medicine has so frequently been mentioned, it is well to state here what is meant by it and the most satisfactory way to give it.

First, give Formulas 2 and 3 (see Chapter I), or composition, adding a teaspoonful of Formula 6; then steam. When in bed repeat the medicine, adding Formula 1, which will cleanse the stomach and assist in keeping up a perspiration. When this has finished operating, give an injection made with the same articles. Where there are symptoms of nervous affection, or spasms, add half a teaspoonful of the nerve powder in each dose given and in the injection. In violent cases, where immediate relief must be had, Formulas 1, 2, 3, and 6 may be given together. Injections may be administered at all times and in all forms of disease to great advantage; *they can do no harm,* and in many instances they are indispensable, especially where there is an inflammatory and morbid state of the bowels, and danger of mortfication. In the last condition, Formula 6 should be added.

Many will consider this heroic treatment. However, it is both harmless and effective. Other and more simple plans of treatment will be outlined as we proceed.

The employment of the steam bath is as desirable as a preventive of sickness as it is in curing it. When a person has been exposed to the cold and is threatened with sickness, it may be prevented, and a long illness and expense saved, by steaming until free perspiration takes place, and at the same time taking the heating medicines such as *Capsicum, pleurisy root,* and *skullcap.*

It is to be noted that if a patient is carried through a course of medicine and steamed, and he has been long under mercurial treatment, then while under the operation of the steam when the heat is at its highest, *the face may swell.* To overcome this, add some vinegar to hot water and soak cloths in this. Wring out dry as possible and apply to swollen parts as hot as can be borne, and also permit the patient to inhale the vinegar fumes. As soon as one cloth cools, apply another hot one, and continue until swelling subsides.

In many instances it may be found inconvenient or even impossible to give the vapor or steam baths. In such cases the bath tub should be half filled with water as warm as the patient can comfortably bear. Immerse the entire body in the water, and permit the patient to remain in it for five to thirty minutes, according to the condition to be overcome. Dry the body well, and give an alcohol rub.

In high temperatures it is the modern practice to use ice caps or packs. This lowers the resistance of the system and is a shock. Vapor and steam baths, as well as immersion, will do all that ice packs can do, and besides it will help to eliminate poisons and congestion and reinforce the vital forces to help them maintain life until the enemy disease is overcome. Immersion is indicated whenever the temperature rises above 101° F. When the temperature reaches 102.5° to 103°

these baths may be given every 5 hours. Care must be exercised to avoid chills. This is readily done by quickly drying the body after leaving the warm water and following this by a rub. In cases where there is extreme weakness, only a part of the body at a time should be bathed with tepid water, and this followed by a rub. The vital forces must be reinforced by natural stimulants such as will be described.

The Pack Bath

In chronic congestions known as tumors and cancers, and in blood diseases such as syphilis and scrofula, as also in wasting diseases such as tuberculosis, the pack bath is preferred. This will gradually draw out all poisons from the system and establish a normal activity —an equilibrium.

A couch without a back is best for the purpose. Spread five to six woolen blankets of large size over this. Dip a linen sheet, which is large enough to cover the body from neck down, feet included, in cold or cool water. The temperature of the water should depend upon the strength of the patient, the ailment, the desired result, and the tolerance to cold applications. Wring the cloth out thoroughly, and wrap around the entire body. The patient now lies down on the covered couch, and first a blanket on one side is drawn up closely over the body, care being taken that the feet are thoroughly wrapped up and the neck tightly tucked in, then a blanket from the other side, and this continued until all blankets are wrapped over the patient. In a few minutes reaction will set in, and the patient will commence to perspire. Give all the cold water or fruit juices desired, and permit the patient to remain until perspiration ceases. Remove the blankets and sheets, give a quick shower or sponge bath, dry off thoroughly, then complete with an alcohol and witch hazel (equal parts) rub. If patient is strong enough, exercise should be taken to cause reaction. If too weak for this, then place in bed and permit him to sleep.

The wet sheet will act as an extra skin and will gradually draw out all poisons from the system. This improves the circulation of the blood. As a result the dead cells, acids and other waste materials are carried off, and new material is carried to the diseased parts for the construction of new cells and tissues.

Dr. August Reinhold said, "The toxins that cause practically all diseases can be eliminated successfully by the wet pack, and any fever can be controlled by this simple application. The body is hot when feverish and, therefore, the cool or cold sheet feels refreshing. It is cooling yet stimulating, and usually the patient falls asleep, and when he awakes the temperature is reduced, and he feels like a new person. Why has the fever left? Because the waste or disease producing materials have been drawn out by the pack, and there is no fuel (congestion) to burn (set up irritation)."

A pack may be given to any part of the body where there is congestion. However, in all conditions where the temperature is above normal the entire body pack should be given. Generally, one pack a day is sufficient, though it may be repeated if necessary to reduce the temperature. Packs may be given in practically all cases where the vapor or steam bath is indicated and is safer and more desirable. As already indicated, it should form part of the treatment in all cases of cancer, tumor, syphilis, scrofula, tuberculosis, and like conditions.

DISEASE

"Disease is a condition that prevents full, free, and regular action. All that is necessary to bring relief and establish order is to remove obstacles to this action and excite the organs to their proper motions. Whatever will invariably, promptly, powerfully and permanently relax, contract, and stimulate will remove all obstructions to vital action and cure all forms of disease is a true medicine. As stimulation is nothing more than rapidly alternating relaxation and contraction (an interchange of activity as in the storage battery), it follows that the two motions in different ways and degrees of rapidity, sometimes relaxing, sometimes contracting with greater or less velocity are all that is necessary."

6.

THE INTERNAL BATH
ALSO KNOWN AS INJECTIONS OR CLYSTERS

This manner of administering medicine (or food) is of the greatest importance in the eradication of disease and the maintaining of strength and will frequently bring relief when all other methods fail.

According to the plans which we have formulated and put into practice for the past fifty years,[1] there are certain objects aimed at in the administration of substances termed medicines for the elimination of disease: to raise the internal heat and maintain it, to promote perspiration, to remove morbid matter from the surface of the mucous membrane, to guard against mortification, and restore the powers of digestion. To best accomplish these objects, the medicines necessary to remove the complaint must be applied to that part where the disease is located. If in the stomach only, then by taking the medicine through the mouth the disease may be reached, but if in the bowels, the same combination should be administered by means of the enema. Whatever is good to eliminate disease when taken into the stomach is doubly beneficial for the same purpose when given by injection, for then it is not changed by the process of ordinary digestion—*the interaction on it of alkalies and acids.* In all cases the grand object is to ceate a natural heat and remove congestions and morbidity.

In all cases of dysentery, colic, piles, and other complaints where the bowels are badly affected, injections should never be dispensed with. It is safe to give them in all cases, and far better that they be given many times, even unnecessarily, than once neglected when actively indicated. In many violent cases, particularly where there is danger of mortification, patients may be treated by administering medicine in this way, when there would be no chance in any other

---

1. This method was one of three; oral medication, direct medication by infusion using the Galvanic current, and in the enema, forming the *International System of Direct Medication.*

way. We, therefore, most seriously advise that these considerations be always borne in mind, and that when quick action is desired the medicated internal bath offers the safest manner.

In many complaints peculiar to women, the internal bath is the most direct means of giving relief. The remedy should be suited to the condition.

The best position is the elbow and knee posture. This permits the easy flow of the medicated water and will reach a greater portion of the mucous membrane of the bowel than any other method. When the greatest amount of activity of the medicine is desired, then it is best first thoroughly to cleanse the bowels by taking a plain internal bath of Castile soap suds using two or more quarts of warm water. After passing this off, the medical mixture may be added to an eighth of a pint of water, injected and retained and absorbed by the mucous membrane directly into the circulation.

Extreme Morbid Conditions

In all extremely morbid conditions, as when there is the formation or accumulation of pus, danger of gangrene or mortification, then one-half ounce of tincture of myrrh and 15 to 30 drops of tincture of *Echinacea* should be added to the quart of warm (not hot) water and this injected into the bowels and helds as long as possible to permit absorption. In the treatment of appendicitis and every other affliction of the alimentary system where there is acute inflammation or congestion which may give rise to inflammation and the formation of pus, this is the ideal treatment. When the affliction is less acute, only the *Echinacea* need be added to the water. These short (2 to 4 ounces of water) enemas may be given as frequently as every hour depending on the severity of the case. If this plan is followed, all food prohibited and only fruit drinks in abundance permitted, then appendicitis will lose its terrors and operations become a rarity except in emergencies.

Ordinary Diarrhoea

In ordinary diarrhœa, whether of adults or infants, the method of procedure is very simple. To a quart of moderately cool (not cold) water, add two tablespoonfuls of tincture of witch hazel and use as an enema. Retain as long as possible to permit absorption and cleansing of the mucous surface. Repeat every one or two hours according to the severity of the case. In children use same proportion of witch hazel with an equal part of water which is to be retained.

If there is a temperature and indication of internal disturbances other than simply diarrhœa, add 15 drops of tincture of purple cone-flowers, and in case where there is a show of pus or blood, a teaspoonful of tincture of myrrh. Tincture of purple cone-flowers controls the pus formation and danger of pus poisoning, and the tincture of myrrh will help to prevent mortification and gangrene. There is no more potent combination than that of witch hazel, myrrh, and purple cone-flowers.

Cathartic Action

To evacuate the bowels, no less than a quart of lukewarm water should be used. Adults may safely take two or even more quarts especially if a long tube is used. To the quart of water add a tablespoonful of dark brown (New Orleans if to be had) sugar, and a very few grains of potassium permanganate, being certain the potassium is completely dissolved. It is best to first add the potassium permanganate being careful that the water is never more than a medium violet in color. The sugar is a relaxant and the potassium permanganate is a splendid antiseptic.

In the case of children only the sugar should be added, and if there is colic in conjunction with the constipation weak catnip tea should be used, to which a small amount of brown sugar has been added. Use only a 1 or 2 ounce rectal (bulb) syringe to avoid the danger of inflating the bowels too much. In all cases where evacuation does not follow within an hour, repeat the enema.

The Enema as a Relaxant

In all conditions where the body is tense and a feverish condition present, no plan of procedure is of greater service than the warm enema. In the beginning of colds and fevers, 15 to 30 drops each of Tinctures of *Asclepias* (Pleurisy Root) and *Eupatorium* (Boneset) and 10 to 30 drops of Tincture *Lobelia,* depending on the severity of the case. When prepared for children, it is best to eliminate the

Lobelia, or to add only one-third the amount. These enemas may be given every hour until equilibrium is established, and the patient rests easily. In convulsions the same formula should be employed, but the strength of the tinctures increased.

The Enema as a Stimulant

In all depressed conditions such as sudden collapse or shock the Thomsonian formula may be used or instead, 10 drops of tincture of *Zingiber* ginger, 5 drops of *Capsicum,* and 15 drops of myrrh to the quart of water. The water should be as hot as can be borne comfortably by the hand, and the enemas repeated every hour until reaction takes place; reaction is usually preceded by a thorough activity of the bowels.

The Enema as a Nervine

In all severe prostrations such as apoplexy, meningitis, lockjaw, and similar conditions, the enema, to which has been added powerful but non-poisonous nervines, is of great importance. Among the very best of these agents is *cypripedium.* To each quart of warm water, 30 to 60 drops of tincture of lady's slipper should be added, and the enema repeated every two to three hours. Where the nervous condition is extreme, 15 drops of the tincture may be added to 3 ounces of water, or even less, and this retained to be absorbed. In appendicitis, when there is great nervousness or irritability, lady's slipper should be added to the enema. Other good nervines may be used instead when it is not procurable.

Antiseptic Enemas

In all conditions where an internal antiseptic is indicated, tincture of purple cone-flowers is the best. If this is to be reinforced, then tincture of myrrh may be added. As already mentioned, potassium permanganate is also a splendid antiseptic but in all but the smallest amount it is a poison. Plain water should never be employed as an enema since it is weakening.

Astringent Enemas

In dysentery, cholera morbus, and like complaints, it is desirable and of great value to administer astringent and tonic enemas. In mild cases, tincture of witch hazel is the choice, or if this is not handy, an infusion of cherry bark will serve as well. When there is danger of, or an indication of pus, tincture of myrrh must be added. In cases where blood is present, 15 to 60 drops of tincture of bayberry must be added. To recapitulate: In ordinary dysentery, tincture of witch hazel in cool water, or cherry bark infusion should be used. When pus is present, however, tincture of myrrh with tincture of witch hazel and even tincture of purple cone-flowers can be used. When blood is present in the stool, all the above is used with the addition of tincture of bayberry. All enemas in cool water and repeated every 1, 2, to 3 hours, according to the severity of the case.

When there is extreme soreness in the bowels, then it is best first to prepare barley water, and to this add the medication. For this purpose the barley should be boiled, and the water carefully passed through a cloth to remove all particles that might irritate the sensitive surface of the bowels.

Nourishing Enemas

In many conditions of the system, and especially in cancer and ulcers of the stomach, in wasting diseases, in unconsciousness and when the stomach refuses to accept food, it is of great value to feed the patient *via* the rectum. First of all, it is necessary to cleanse the rectum by giving an enema composed of warm water and Tincture *Echinacea* to which also has been added 3 drops of Tincture *Capsicum*. After this has been voided, then barley or oatmeal water with the white of an egg well beaten and filtered may be injected and retained to be absorbed. The amount should be no greater than 3 ounces at a time and this may be repeated every $2\frac{1}{2}$ hours. Beef broth, malted milk, milk in which Irish moss has been boiled, or any other nourishing food, which can be liquified and filtered, may be given.

In anemic conditions it is of utmost importance to boil vegetables in water, and then boil down this water to one-third the quantity, and inject this so that the organic mineral elements may be absorbed and help establish equilibrium.

Important Note

Practically every disease may be treated and every organic remedy utilized *via* the rectum, and in most instances, the response is quicker and more favorable than when medication is orally taken. This procedure (singly or in combination, in 2 teaspoons, 4 ounces of water) may be known as direct medication and thoroughly covered in texts of that title.

7.

THE NATURA SYSTEM
(ORIGINALLY KNOWN AS THE
THOMSONIAN SYSTEM)

The original formulary of medication as taught by Dr. Samuel Thomson is first given. Followed by the more modern practices of the eclectic, physiomedical and later Natura physicians. Investigation clearly indicates that in the more rural districts when it is often difficult to obtain the services of a physician, or where the people still have the original faith in nature's remedies, they continue to follow the original Thomsonian system with some modification, because the eight formulas can be prepared in advance and are at hand for immediate use.

First we will discuss Lobelia, the most important agent of the Thomsonian system and its eight formulas.

INDIAN TOBACCO
Lobelia Inflata

The present newly awakening interest in organic medicines made from vegetables, herbs, roots and barks, and more especially Indian tobacco, requires that a more complete description be given than in the original book based on the teachings of the Thomsonian, eclectic physiomedical and/or Natura school, in the present edition.

Common Names: Lobelia, emetic herb (Thomson), pike weed, gagroot, vomitroot.

Parts: Leaves, tops, and seeds.

Preparation: Tincture or infusions.

Dose: Adults: 10 to 60 drops; children, 3 to 20 drops.

Average Dose: 10 to 30 drops minimum of tincture of 10 per cent drug strength.

Recognized Specific Indications

Angina pectoris, apoplexy, asthma, bronchitis, croup, infantile convulsions, epilepsy, diphtheria, hemorrhagic diphtheria, dysmenorrhea, acute heart attacks, heatstroke, hysteria, migraine, ovarian spasms, intestine spasms, spinal meningitis, tetanus, tonsillitis, whooping cough.

Symptomatic Indications

In short, labored breathing, sense of suffocation; dyspnoea; precordial oppression; pain in chest of heavy, sore, or oppressive character; dry cough, either with scant or over secretions; asthmatic seizures; short, lacinating pain radiating from the heart center to left shoulder and arm; spasmodic muscular contraction; muscular rigidity; infantile convulsions due to some form of internal irritation; hysterical convulsion; rigid os uteri accompaned by rigid rim; perineal and vaginal rigidity during labor, angina pectoris.

ACTION

The action of *Lobelia* is upon the central nervous system and the sympathic nerve ganglia. It is generally classed as a gastro-intestinal irritant because in sufficiently large doses it produces emesis.[1] The action of small doses is upon the cardiac area slowing heart action and is followed generally by a more or less accelerated pulse. The action of small, frequent doses (as indicated) is to stimulate; of large doses to relax first and then followed by stimulation to the organic action. Small doses stimulate digestion, the secretions, and poor circulation, especially when due to enervated states. When *Lobelia* is combined with other appropriate remedies, its tendency is to establish normalcy of the entire system and stimulate all the organs of the body; hence it is of great benefit in all chronic or semi-chronic conditions. In acute ailments, such as acute indigestion, the onset of diphtheria, croup, scarlet fever, smallpox, tetanus or the bites of poisonous insects where immediate effect is imperative, doses large enough to produce emesis should be given, to be followed by small doses in combination with such stimulants as *Capsicum*.

---

1. Our experience with Lobelia does *not* bear out this conclusion. Improper use of any drug may produce undesirable symptoms.

In angina pectoris, neuralgia of the heart, and pulmonary apoplexy, doses of 20 drops should be given and repeated as necessary. It is a cardiac stimulant and acts as a sedative. In markedly slow pulse-wave, *Lobelia* in small frequent doses is *the* remedy; it is indicated in all full, oppressed, or sluggish pulses, especially if associated with precordial oppression, thoracic pain, difficulty in breathing, soreness of chest, nausea and coated tongue, and fullness of tissue.

In obstetrical cases, *Lobelia* relaxes muscular rigidity and readily overcomes *rigis os* during parturition, and also relaxes the perineal tissues protecting the parts against lacerations.

In loss of appetite and slow digestion, this agent is of great value. It is best given in small doses and may be combined with other indicated agents. It is decidedly valuable in the atonic types of indigestion and dyspepsia associated with sick headache due to gastric disturbances; in such cases it is best given in small frequent doses. In chronic respiratory disorders it increases or decreases the secretions according to the dosage. In dry, barking, or hacking coughs, where mucous rales are heard and there is difficulty in raising the sputum, *Lobelia* is most valuable, and is equally serviceable in chronic coughs if combined with other indicated agents. It is of great service in the coughs of measles where sluggish circulation is present and eruptions are slow to appear or fail to fully develop. In scarlet fever and measles, *Lobelia* causes determination of the blood to the skin, promotes tardy eruptions, and helps reestablish natural balance when dangerous retrocession occurs for some reason. In whooping cough, where secretions of a stringy character have a strangling effect on the sufferer, it should be given in small frequent doses. *Lobelia* is an invaluable agent in all stages of la grippe and epidemic influenza. It is a vital stimulant, regulates imperfect circulation, and controls cough and expectoration.

LOBELIA EXTERNALLY

Lobelia is a valuable ingredient in *all* forms of poultices where relaxation is desired. Infusions or alcoholic extracts may be used or powdered substituted. It well combines with flax-seed or slippery elm in the relief of insect bites, bruises and sprains and of various pains. Powdered *Lobelia* is well combined with lard and applied warm in acute thoracic diseases or any form of soreness of the chest.

Lobelia in any form may be effectively combined with other agents and used as a poultice in the pains and inflammation present in pneumonia, broncho-pneumonia, bronchitis, croup, pleurisy, acute pharyngitis, tonsillitis, orchitis, ovaritis, arthritis, inflammatory rheumatism, and for all localized pains in the joint and muscular structures.

Personal Remarks

The number *one* agent on the *Natura* physician's armamentarium is *Lobelia*. *Lobelia* is one of Nature's few *dual* agents in the relief of human ailments. It is both a relaxant and a stimulant; depending altogether on how it is prescribed, hence if the *Natura* physician had to choose one remedy from all others, it would be *Lobelia* and he could practice successfully. So many claims have been made for this agent, and so many more could be *honestly* made for it, were its virtues fully understood. Most unfortunately it has been called a *quack* remedy, and most *unjustly, Lobelia* has been, and continues to be—labeled a *poison*.[2] If this is to indicate that an unlimited amount may not be prescribed without harmful reactions then such labelling is justified, otherwise not. In an experience of fifty-six years (at the writing) I have prescribed it for children and people advanced in age; in amounts of three drops to new born children; fifteen drops every fifteen minutes for hours, or maximum doses of 60 drops, to older persons with never any but the best results. I have given it where immediate relaxation was an absolute necessity to be followed by a stimulating effect, and it has not failed me. If there were such a thing as a general panacea, I would say that *Lobelia* comes nearer to being such than any other agent I have used in all of these many years.

The Experience with Indian Tobacco of Practicing Physicians of Renown—

Ellingwood, of Chicago, internationally recognized as an authority, gives Indian tobacco a foremost place in the treatment of many cases of disease such as angina pectoris, anuria, apoplexy, asthma,

---

2. The pharmacy law of Pennsylvania requires that any drug that may be considered deleterious to normal health in doses of 1 fluid dram or 60 grains by weight *must be labeled "poison."*

Merck's *Index,* Seventh Edition, does *not* cite *Lobelia* either as a quack remedy or a poison, simply as an expectorant or an emetic in large doses.

bronchitis, pneumonia, croup, infantile convulsions, diphtheria, hemorrhagic diphtheria, dysmenorrhea, epilepsy, acute heart failure, heatstroke, hysteria, migraine, rigid os, ovarian pains, spasms in the intestines, spinal meningitis, tetanus, tonsillitis, tuberculosis, whooping cough.

Not long ago because of misconceptions relative to Indian tobacco, its value and proper use, many physicians would not have had the courage to use it as much as the most ethical physicians do today. The following item, which appeared in the public press, will be of interest to Natura and all liberal physicians.

"Heart Action Had Stopped When Surgeon Injected Fluid."

Baltimore, Md., July 22, 1925.—A new-born baby, given up for dead, now lives, and is thriving as a result of an injection of lobelin solution.

Dr. Walter Cox, of the Franklin Square Hospital, injected the drug, the operation being described as involving great risk.

Lobelin is derived from Lobelia inflata, a form of a large common blue flower which, for a century, has been known as a heart stimulant.

"We could not start the baby's breathing," Dr. Cox said. "Finally, we concluded it was dead. There seemed to be no way to revive life. Its heart had stopped beating.

"Since I was convinced the baby was dead there was nothing to fear in using the drug. I plunged the hypodermic into the baby and almost immediately it started to breathe, and heart action was restored. This marks the opening of a new avenue in obstetrics."

There is nothing *new* in this. Dr. Samuel Thomson used *Lobelia* —in the infusion form—for the same purpose (restoration of suspended animation) almost from the very beginning of his practice, and was wholesomely condemned for using such a "deadly poison." Eclectic and physio-medical physicians have used *Lobelia* consistently in powder, tincture, and hypodermic form and without a single recorded fatality.

Tablets: 1 to 60 grains. In chronic conditions, 1 to 5 grains together with 1 or 2 grains of *Capsicum* is the approved dosage. In acute cases, 15 to 60 grains may be safely given and repeated in 30 to 60 minutes. The larger doses should not be given except in an emergency when the aid of a physician is not to be had.

Tincture: Specifics only should be prescribed. The dosage is the same as for the tablet.

Hypodermically: To be used only by physicians, and seldom in other than acute cases.

To disabuse the mind of the laity as to the danger of *Lobelia* we cite the following cases:

"A girl, thirteen years old, took a violent chill and soon became unconscious. Instead of resorting to the usual remedies I gave her 30 minims of *Lobelia* and wrapped her in a hot blanket. In half an hour she regained consciousness. An hour later she was again unconscious. I then gave her 60 minims *Lobelia*. In half an hour she began to show much warmth and commenced to sweat profusely. She recovered promptly. I have used *Lobelia* perhaps a hundred times in congested chills, and when it seemed that the patient was at death's door. Results have been uniform."—*A. W. B.*, M.D.

"In a case of scarlet fever, with complications, *Lobelia* proved of the greatest benefit. General dropsy appeared; breathing was difficult, pulse almost imperceptible. Little hope for recovery. I gave a hypodermic of 30 minims of *Lobelia*. In forty minutes, 40 drops more. In one hour another 30 drops, after which I could see some change for the better. In the afternoon she was was much better; she was warm, pulsation at the wrist weak, but plainly found. There was great improvement in breathing. Next morning the patient was much better and resting. Convalescence was slow but continuous and in the end complete."—*E. H.*, M.D.[3]

3. *The Gleaner,* September, 1925.

When emesis (vomiting) is sought, 15 to 30 grains or as many as 50 grains, *Lobelia* in tablet form, or that many drops of the tincture, should be given in water of the body temperature. If vomiting does not follow within a very short time, give half a cup of water of the same temperature every 5 minutes until emesis does occur, then follow immediately with 3 to 5 grains of *Capsicum* every half hour until three doses have been taken, and then the remedy indicated by the condition.

According to Drs. Thomson, Scudder, Lyle, Greer, Stephens and modern Natura physicians:

Lobelia is indicated when the pulse is full and oppressed, or small and feeble, oppression in the precordium, labored action of the heart, cardiac (heart) pain, oppression of the chest with difficult and labored respiration and the accumulation of mucous in the bronchial tubes.

Lobelia is a specific in most cases of angina pectoris and neuralgia of the heart. It is the indicated remedy when the patient complains of oppression in the chest and difficult breathing. It is the remedy in laryngitis in both children and adults. It is directly indicated in all conditions where there is a morbid congestion of the mucous membranes. *Lobelia* is one of the most direct and valuable stimulants to the sympathetic nervous system, and it favorably influences every organ and function supplied or controlled by these nerves.

Where there is lack of vitality to combat the invasion of disease, *Lobelia* is always indicated.

Lobelia is dual in its activity. In small doses it stimulates. In large doses it relaxes and *must be followed* by a stimulant such as *Capsicum*.

In all conditions of congestion, wherever they may be, *Lobelia*, due to its influence on the blood vessels, lessens the depression through the vaso-motor, and strengthens the muscular action of the vessel walls which propel the blood onward, overcoming the condition.

For spasms in children, *Lobelia* is the ideal remedy. It will give quick relief, after which the cause must be sought and relieved by the indicated remedies.

In whooping-cough, false heart spasms, spasmodic coughs, and many forms of asthma, it is the ideal remedial agent.

Lobelia is a powerful anti-spasmodic acting on the nerve and respiratory centers, thereby improving oxygenation of the blood.

In the convulsions of childhood, as in all other forms of convulsion, it should be the first remedy given.

In pnuemonia and all other conditions of the congestion of the lungs when breathing is difficult and painful, the pulse rapid, and the expression of the countenance drawn, *Lobelia* is the first remedy to be given to induce relaxation and equalize the circulation of the blood, thereby removing the congestions.

On the contrary, when the circulation is feeble, the extremities cold, face pallid, and there is oppression, it is equally efficient with the aid of *Capsicum* to restore normalcy.

In all cases of zymotic (inner filth) diseases such as scarlet fever, chickenpox, measles, and smallpox it is of supreme importance. First, a large dose to cleanse the stomach of poisonous matter, then in conjunction with other remedies cleanse the entire system of congestions and establish equilibrium.

Lobelia acts directly upon the regulating centers of the system (thus its influence to establish equilibrium), those of heart, circulation, nervous system and digestive organs. It supports the heart, overcomes excessive blood pressure in any portion of the body, and restores interaction between the functions of the various organs.

Lobelia is a restorative to the nerve force at the several centers, acts directly upon the heart and the lungs, restores the resisting potency of every center to the invasion of disease, and establishes harmony between the nervous and circulatory systems.

When the heart is weak, *Lobelia* is a restorative, and following its use the pulse becomes strong and natural.

In the dreaded diphtheria, *Lobelia* hypodermically given is of greater potency, and in every sense far more valuable, not to mention being more natural, than almost any other agent.

In all bronchial difficulties, whether asthma, croup, or pneumonia, Lobelia should be given in a relaxant dose—sufficient to cause free vomiting and thus cleanse the stomach and then be given as part of the aftertreatment.

In epilepsy and all other contractive ailments, *Lobelia* should be given first in doses large enough to cleanse the stomach and relax the system, and then be followed by corrective treatment. Spasms, whether of the chest, spine, muscles, or sex organs should be treated in the same manner.

In many forms of digestive disturbances, *Lobelia* is an ideal remedy. This is especially true in nervous dyspepsia where there is a feeling more of nausea than of pain, an oppressive feeling, like a dead weight, after eating. Also, in those conditions where there is a feeling of coldness, or a faintness at the pit of the stomach. In such conditions, a few grains of *Lobelia* and an equal amount of *Capsicum* (tablet form) may be taken directly after eating. In acute indigestion, a condition which has killed countless people and where the verdict has nearly always been "heart failure," *Lobelia* given in a dose sufficiently large to promptly empty the stomach will hardly, if ever, fail. It is the one agent that one may safely rely upon. It should always be followed by a stimulant and nervine.

Lobelia is essential in labor. It will allay and regulate the violent pains in the loins during labor due to rigidity of the passages, and is far safer and much to be preferred to ergot or other agents generally employed.

In disorders of the menstrual period, it is, with the addition of such agents as pennyroyal, the ideal agent to relieve contraction and pain and establish normalcy.

In hysteria, whether due to congested ovaries, swollen uterus, or other cause *Lobelia* with nervines may be safely relied upon to bring relief.

Important: Whether *Lobelia* is given in the powdered, tinctural, or tablet form (most desirable when given alone), it is always to be remembered that the full dose should be given at once. If emesis does not occur promptly, follow with slightly warm water every 5 minutes until there is free vomiting. This plan is followed in all cases where emptying of the stomach and relaxation is desired, as in spasms, congestions, fits, and infectious diseases. As soon as the vomiting ceases, stimulants and nervines must be given.

When stimulation is desired, then the dose is always small, from one to five grains in conjunction with a stimulant such as *Capsicum*.

These instructions follow closely the original. The various herbal agents are fully described in the chapter on family and household remedies.

Formula One, The Emetic—*Lobelia*

1. The powdered leaves and pods. This is the most common form of using it; and from one-half to a teaspoon may be taken in warm water, sweetened; or the same quantity may be added to either of the other numbers when taken to cleanse the stomach, overpower a cold, and promote a free perspiration.

2. A tincture made from the green herb. This is used to counteract the effects of poison (taken either internally or applied externally) and for asthma and other complaints of the lungs. For a dose, add a grain or two of *Capsicum* in a half teacup of warm water, sweetened, and in all cases of nerve affection add one-half teaspoon of nerve powder. For the external effects of poison, take the above dose with the tincture, and bathe the parts affected, repeating until relieved.

3. The seeds reduced to a fine powder and mixed with Formulas 2 and 6, is for the most violent attacks of spasms and other complaints, such as lockjaw, bite of dog with hydrophobia, fits, and in all cases of suspended animation where the vital spark is nearly extinct. For a dose, give a teaspoonful, and repeat till relief is obtained; then follow with a tea made of No. 3 for canker.

For children, the dose must be regulated according to their age. If very young, steep a quarter of a teaspoonful of the powder in half a teacupful of warm water, or in a tea made with raspberry leaves, and give a teaspoonful of the tea at a time. First strain through a cloth, and sweeten, repeat the dose every 15 minutes until it operates. Give pennyroyal or other herb tea, for a drink.

4. Tablets may be substituted for the herb. Ten to 15 grains in one-half cup of warm water every 15 minutes until the stomach has been completely relieved of all its contents.

Lobelia will do quickly all that the stomach pump can do and do it as efficiently and with better results.

Formula Two—Cayenne Pepper (*Capsicum*)

Nature's stimulant without any reaction, Cayenne pepper is the most pronounced natural stimulant in the entire *materia medica*. It cannot be equalled by any other known agent where a powerful and prolonged stimulant is called for as in congestive chills, heart failure, and other conditions calling for quick action. The entire circulation is affected by this agent, and there is no reaction. In this it stands alone as ideal.

In congested, ulcerated, or infectious sore throat it is an excellent agent, but should be combined with myrrh to relieve and remove the morbidity.

Cayenne pepper is antiseptic, and therefore a most valuable agent as a gargle in ordinary sore throat or diphtheria.

In uterine hemorrhages it is ideal combined with bayberry and will do more than any other remedy could.

Cayenne pepper has the power to arouse the action of the secreting organs and always follows the use of Indian tobacco.

When there is inactivity of the entire system, as in "spring fever," Cayenne pepper is indicated. In fact, whenever there is disinclination to activity it is an ideal stimulant, arousing the sluggish organism to action.

In indigestion where gas is present, it should be given in conjunction with small doses (1 to 5 grains) of Indian tobacco. Cayenne pepper increases the glandular activity of both stomach and intestines.

In all so-called "low" fevers where the temperature is subnormal, Cayenne pepper is indicated and should be prescribed consistently.

At the onset of a cold, when there are chills, cold, and clammy feelings, the feet damp and cold, Cayenne pepper should be taken in full dose (5 to 10 grains). In these cases Cayenne pepper is more efficient than quinine and there is no reaction—no undesirable after-effect.

Even in cholera morbus and atonic diarrhoea where stimulants are usually contraindicated, Cayenne pepper is valuable in that it "tones" up the organs and establishes natural activity.

In all diseases prostrating in their nature, whether pneumonia, pleurisy, or typhoid fever, Cayenne pepper is invaluable in the prescription as the toning agent which helps the system to throw off the disease and reestablish equilibrium.

In all acute conditions where Cayenne pepper is indicated, the call is for the maximum dose—from 3 to 10 grains, preferably in tablet form—followed by a large drink of hot water. In chronic and sluggish conditions, the small dose frequently given is 1 to 3 grains with either hot or cold water.

Cayenne pepper plasters are valuable in pneumonia, pleurisy, and other acute congestions. Combine with Indian tobacco and bran or hops. One hour is the maximum time to keep them applied.

Formula Three—The Canker Remedy

Combine Bayberry root bark, white pond lily root, and the inner bark of hemlock equal parts, and pound them well, mix thoroughly; steep 1 ounce of the powder in a pint of boiling water and give a common wineglassful (2 to 4 tablespoons) sweetened for a dose.

Note: It is desirable to have this preparation always on hand and ready for use. To do this, take 1 ounce of the powder, add to a quart of water and boil until it is reduced to 1 pint. Strain, sweeten with honey, and add 3 ounces of grain alcohol. This will keep indefinitely. When needed, add one-half wineglass to a cup of hot water.

If the ingredients suggested cannot be had, substitute sumach bark, leaves or berries, red raspberry or witch hazel leaves, marsh rosemary, or either of the other articles mentioned before. This may be prepared in the same manner.

When the violence of the disease requires a course of medicine add 5 grains of Formula Two, 15 grains of Formula One, and an equal amount of Formula Eight. This dose is to be given three times at intervals of 15 minutes, and the same combination in a quart of warm water, as the internal bath. This course of medicine may be repeated if found necessary. If mortification is known to exist, suspected or feared, a teaspoonful of Formula Six, may be added to the combination for internal bath.

After the patient has recovered sufficiently from the operation of the medicine, which is usually in 2 or 3 hours, give the steam or pack bath. This is heroic treatment and indicated in severe illness, and when the aid of a physician is not to be secured. It is in no sense a dangerous procedure and in many instances will save life.

This operation is sufficient for one time and must be repeated each day, or every other day, as the circumstances of the case require until the disorder is removed. Three times will generally be sufficient, and sometimes once or twice will answer the purpose, but in severe cases it may be necessary to continue to carry the sufferer through a regular course two or three times a week, for a considerable length of time.

After the patient has been taken through a course of the medicine, great care must be taken to keep up an internal heat, so as to produce perspiration by giving occasionally Formula Two or the composition powder.

During the period of treatment give milk porridge or gruel, well-seasoned with cayenne pepper. In cases where the liver is at fault, clam broth should be the only food given during the entire course of the treatment.

A teacup of the tea of Formula Two, should be given night and morning to prevent a relapse and during the day a tea made of poplar bark. If constipation exists, a tea of bitter root.

As soon as the disorder is under control, give bitters, Formula Four, to correct the bile and restore the digestion; and half a wineglass of the syrup of Formula Five, two or three times a day which will strengthen the stomach and assist in regulating the digestive organism and its functions.

These instructions are to be followed only in the more violent attacks of disease and such as have become settled. Among these are apoplexy, severe cases of asthma, bronchitis, pneumonia, croup, and convulsions which require heroic treatment. Diphtheria, ovarian and uterine cramps, spasms, meningitis and tetanus, and in tuberculosis where all other treatment has failed.

FORMULA FOUR—BITTERS

Bitter herb, or balmony, barberry and poplar bark equal parts, pulverized, 1 ounce of the mixed powder added to a pint of boiling water, and steep for one-half hour. Filter, and add one-half pint of grain alcohol. Dose: a tablespoon in hot water every few hours. Where stimulation is necessary, 3 grains of cayenne pepper is to be added to each dose as taken.

These bitters will help correct the bile and restore a natural appetite by improving the digestion. It may be freely used as a preventative of disease and a restorative after illness.

FORMULA FIVE—SYRUP

Poplar bark and the root of bayberry, 1 pound each. Ground or powder, and boil slowly in a gallon of water for one-half hour; strain and add 4 pounds of sugar or 5 pounds of honey. Bring to a boil and skim. Add one-half pound of either ground peach stone meats or cherry stone meats. When cool, add 1 quart of good brandy and bottle for future use. Dosage: one-half a wineglass, two or three times a day. A smaller amount may be prepared by observing the same proportions.

This syrup is of exceptional value to strengthen the action of stomach and bowels, and to restore vitality during and after an illness. By using this syrup in combination with Formula Three in the first stage of dysentery, it will generally bring quick relief.

FORMULA SIX—SPECIAL DROPS

Formula Six is made by combining one-half gallon of good brandy, or one gallon of first class wine, one-half pound of powdered gum myrrh, 1 ounce of Formula Two, all heated in a stone jug to 140° drained and bottled.

These drops are prescribed and of great benefit where pain is present in morbid conditions which might result in mortification. One or 2 teaspoons of the drops may be given alone, or the same quantity added to the dose of any of the medicines previously mentioned. They may also be used to bathe external swellings or morbid sores. It has proven an excellent remedy in rheumatism when taken internally and applied externally; and depended on as a household remedy for bruises, sprains, swollen joints, and old sores, as well as to allay inflammation, reduce swellings, ease pain, and create a tendency to healing old sores. In the application of Formula Six for sprains and bruises, it is well to add gum camphor.

In modern practice, the Natura and liberal physician substitutes tincture of coneflower, 5 to 30 drops is the ideal and dependable remedy in all acute septic infections. In septicemia (blood poisoning), in the bites of poisonous snakes and insects, in gangrenous conditions and malignant ulceration, in peritonitis and morbid conditions of the bowels, such as are present in typhoid fever, cholera morbus, and cholera infantum, it is the one remedy that does not disappoint.

Tincture of myrrh: For external applications in cold sores, gangrene, and all forms of poisoning and morbidity, myrrh is the indicated remedy and may be applied freely without dilution. Dose 3 to 5 drops also may be added to purple coneflowers for internal use.

Formula Seven—Composition Powder

Two pounds of bayberry root bark, 1 pound of the inner bark of hemlock, 1 pound of ginger, 2 ounces of Cayenne pepper, 2 ounces of cloves, all pounded fine and sifted through a fine sieve and well mixed together. For a dose, a teaspoon of the powder in one-half teacup of boiling water; permitted to stand until sufficiently cool, strained, then 1 tablespoon of honey added, patient put to bed or in a pack bath, and the remedy given.

This remedy is ideal in the first stages of diseases such as colds, chills, and fevers. It is a remedy of great value, and may be given safely in all complaints of men, women and children, and it will prevent, at the onset, the greater part of acute diseases.

It is excellent to relax (in dysentery), pain in the stomach and bowels and to remove obstructions caused by cold or loss of inward heat and vitality. By taking a dose on retiring and applying a hot water bottle or electric pad to the feet, it will ward off or cure a cold; and repeated several times quickly, will cut short an attack of pleurisy and other lung affections. When the symptoms are violent, with much pain, add to each dose a teaspoon of Formula Six, and 5 grains of Formula One. In nervous symptoms add one-half teaspoon of the nerve powder, and in giving an internal bath do likewise. In very severe attacks, and where the services of a good physician cannot be had, a regular course of medicine should be given.

Formula Eight—Nerve Powder

American valerian or lady's slipper. This is sometimes called umbil, or male and female nervines.

There are four species of this valuable vegetable, one male and three females. The male is called yellow umbil, and grows in swamps and wet lands. It has a large cluster of fibrous roots matted together joined to a solid root, which puts forth several stalks that grow about 2 feet high; it has leaves resembling the poke leaf. The female varieties are distinguished by the color of the blossoms, which are red, red and white, and white. The red has but two leaves which grow out of the ground, and lean over to the right and left, between which a single stalk shoots up to a height of from 8 to 10 inches bearing on its top a red blossom of a very singular form that gives it the name of female umbil. This kind is found on high ledges and swamps. The red and white and white umbils grow only in swamps, and is in larger clusters of roots than the yellow, but in a similar form; its top is similar to the red, except the color of the blossom. The yellow and red are the best for medicine; the roots should be dug in the fall when done growing, or in the spring, before the tops put forth. If dug when growing, the roots will nearly all dry up. When the roots are dug, they must be washed clean, carefully dried, and then ground into a powder, sifted through a fine sieve and preserved from the air for future use.

This powder is composed of the best of known nervines. It will produce the most beneficial effects in all cases of nervous affections, as also in hysterical symptoms. It is perfectly harmless and may be used in all cases of disease with safety; and is much better than the dangerous and habit forming narcotics which number their victims by the millions. This powder has a tendency to promote sleep and is highly soothing, but this is due to its potency to quiet the nerves and to create a state of ease, permitting sleep during which naure may tone up the system and heal the afflictions. One-half a teaspoon may be given in hot water and the dose repeated as often as necessary. The same quantity may be mixed with doses of any of the other numbers and also used in the internal bath. In general practice the tinctures should be substituted.

NATURAL MAN

Under the natural plan or—if you wish—the Divine plan, man continues strong, well, and virile by supplying his body with the elements and *only* such which it requires to maintain a balance—an equilibrium (health being equilibrium). All these elements are obtainable from the organic (organized) kingdoms, principally the vegetables (this term includes all herbs). As indicated by biblical authority, what have been known as herbs are actually vegetables—foods that supply the body with required elements to maintain a balance. Fruits, nuts, cereals, and even eggs, milk, and cheese come under this classification. The latter—milk, cheese, and eggs—are merely *pre*-digested and highly organized (vitalized) vegetables, fruits, and cereals, having been consumed and converted by an animal organism.

8.

THE NATURA PHYSICIAN'S ARMAMENTARIUM

The agents and prescriptions, the effectiveness of which have been thoroughly tested by Thomsonian, Eclectic, Physio-Medical, and during the last 50 years, by *Natura* Physicians.

Both the minimum and maximum dosage of the single agent and each agent in the prescription is given. *It is generally best, except in emergencies, that the physician start with the minimum dose.* In all instances, dosage should be graduated according to age and symptoms.

BARBERRY, COMMON

Berberis Aquifolium Vulgaris

Common names: Oregon Grape, Mountain Grape.

Barberry is a common herb because its red berries have been used by housewives in preserving certain foods. Its bark, the only part used in medicine, is intensely bitter and has been known as one of the "old woman's" medicines because of its general use in infusion as a stomach and liver agent.

Because it is so intensely bitter, *the dosage should be small,* though there have been no reports of harmful results following its almost universal use as a stomach bitters.

The natura physician uses it chiefly in the relief of torpid conditions of the liver and in very small doses for the spleen. It is indicated in all placid conditions of the stomach, but should be used only in chronic condition. Country people, not having easy access to physicians, gathered the herb, added a portion, usually not measured, but generally about 2 ounces to a quart of good whiskey, permitted it to steep for 3 or 4 days, then took a tablespoon of it before meals. This we find, on investigation, is still continued in many families.

In jaundice, accompanied by loss of strength and poor appetite, it is valuable. It is likewise of good service in malarial diseases (where Quinine cannot be had or is counter indicated) when combined with such remedies as *Capsicum, Lobelia* and *Hydrastis,* these agents modifying its more drastic influence. A small proportion may be added with benefit to all preparations for stomach and liver conditions.

In the early stages of tuberculosis it is of much value if combined with:

Tincture of Goldenseal (*Hydrastis canadensis*)	7 to 10 drops
Tincture of Barberry (*Berberis vulgaris*)	3 to 7 drops
Tincture of Cayenne Pepper (*Capsicum frutescens*) or (*Capsicum minimum*)	2 to 4 drops

Dosage: According to condition and age.

This same combination is excellent in catarrhal conditions of the upper passages leading to the lungs, and as a tonic in weak and debilitated conditions of the system, and in convalescence following serious illness.

Dosage of the tincture *Berberis* alone, 3 to 4 times a day in water.

BAYBERRY

Myrica Cerifera

Common names: Myrtle, Wax Myrtle, Candle Berry, Waxberry.

In foulness of the mucous membranes, it is by some considered even superior to Myrrh. It is more pleasant to take and not as harsh in its action; useful and indicated where Myrrh might be considered as too active.

In scrofulous diarrhoea, chronic cholera and goitre, *Myrica* is one of the best agents.

Its influence on the uterus is very *positive,* and for this reason it is the one dependable remedy in uterine hemorrhages, whether due to abortion, miscarriage, or any other cause. Fifteen to 60 drops every 15 to 60 minutes, depending on the severity of the condition, is the dose. The uterus also may be packed with cotton saturated with this tincture.

In *prolapsus uteri* it is splendid, and *in parturition it cannot well be excelled*. It induces better contractions, and when given near the end of the confinement *it will anticipate flooding,* and should there be excessive lochia it will assist in stopping the excess. Its influence is also good in controlling the flow during menstruation and hemorrhages from other parts of the body and is a valuable agent in the treatment of female complaints.

In hot infusions or tincture in hot water, it gradually arouses the circulation and favors an outward flow of blood; a free perspiration, so desirable in many high temperatures will generally follow, and this will be even more abundant, if *Zingaber* is added:

Tincture of Bayberry (*Myrica cerifera*)	10 to 20 drops
Tincture of Ginger (*Zingiber officinale*)	8 to 15 drops

In water three times a day.

When the stomach is very foul in conjunction with *Lobelia,* it will be useful as an emetic, which is very desirable in all cases where this condition is present; as well as in conditions frequently present in mercurial cachexia, acrofula, and secondary syphilis:

Tincture of Bayberry (*Myrica cerifera*)	10 to 20 drops
Tincture of Indian Tobacco (*Lobelia inflata*)	3 to 10 drops

In hot water every 15 minutes until emesis.

Dosage of tincture of *Myrica* alone 10 to 30 drops in water as indicated.

"*Myrica* is both a general and special stimulant to the mucous membranes. It is one of the few astringents which does not provoke a rise in temperature. Increased flow of mucous, whether in bronchopulmonic disease, sore throat, or disease of the stomach or bowels calls for its action. It *aids digestion, nutrition, and blood-making,* and is useful in chronic gastritis, muco-enteritis, chronic catarrhal diarrhoea, atonic leucorrhoea, and dysentery with typhoid symptoms. It is a useful stimulant in typhoid and other low fevers, and is indicated particularly in the sore throat of scarlet fever, when the tissues are feeble and swollen. It is indicated in feeble circulation, useful in in sore throat, sore mouth, sore and bleeding gums when spongy and flabby."—*Dr. Wilmeth—Lloyd.*

BEARBERRY

Arctostaphylos Uva-Ursi

Common names: Upland Cranberry, Arberry.

Best known as *the diabetes remedy.* Uva Ursi is especially astringent and tonic depending upon these qualities for the most of its good effects. It is particularly useful in chronic diarrhoea, dysentery, profuse menstruation, piles, diabetes, and other similar complaints. It possesses rare curative principles when administered for diseases of the urinary organs, more especially in chronic affections of the kidneys, mucous discharges from the bladder, inflammation of this organ, and all derangements of the urinary passages. It is also a valuable assistant in the cure of gonorrhoea of long standing, gleet, whites (*fluor albus*), ulceration of the *cervix uteri,* pain in the vesical region. Many physicians rely upon *Uva Ursi* as the basis of their treatment for gonorrhoea, when accompanied by mucous discharges, and for kindred afflictions. Its tannic and gallic acid give it great power in rectifying and extirpating the obstinate and disagreeable complaints mentioned.

Uva Ursi is best combined with *Populus:*

Tincture of Upland Cranberry (*Arctostaphylos Uva-Ursi*	10 to 20 drops
Tincture of Quaking Aspen (*Populus tremuloides*)	2 to 15 drops

Dosage: Three or more times a day either in hot or cold water depending on desired effects.

Dosage: Tincture of *Uva Ursi* alone, 10 to 20 drops in water 3 or 4 times a day.

When given in the treatment of diabetes, *Vaccinum Myrtillus* should be combined with it:

Tincture of Upland Cranberry (*Arctostaphylos Uva-Ursi*)	10 to 20 drops
Tincture of Blueberry leaves (*Vaccinum myrtillus*)	20 to 40 drops

In water 3 or more times a day.

In domestic use the procedure was to cover the leaves of either or both with 3 times the amount of the Bearberry leaves with good brandy, permit to infuse for a week, then add a teaspoonful to a cup of the infusion.

BEARSFOOT, AMERICAN

Polymnia Uvedalia

Common names: Leaf Cup, Balsamic resin.

Called the mammitis remedy. There are not too many natural agents indicated in this condition, *Uvedalia,* therefore, should be in the medicine case of every *Natura* physician.

It is an alternative and stimulant. The liver, spleen, and stomach are greatly influenced by this agent.

The important influence of *Uvedalia* is in the treatment of *non-*malignant, indurated swellings, such as mammitis and enlarged (engorged) cervical nodules.

Dosage: Tincture of *Uvedalia alone,* 10 to 25 drops, three or more times a day. Dosage and frequency depend on condition for which it is prescribed.

BITTER ROOT

Apocynum Androsaemifolium

Common name: Bitter Root.

Often called the gall-stone remedy.

The root is extremely bitter and is considered one of the best correctors of the bile; equal, if not of greater value than bile usually given for this purpose. It is of much value in correcting costiveness producing, as it generally does, natural bowel movement. Given in large doses, it will act as a cathartic or as an emetic often desirable in jaundice. It is a splendid substitute for *Lobelia* as an emetic for those who are still under the impression that *Lobelia* is a poison.

In jaundice, gall-stones, and chronic sluggish conditions of the liver, Bitter Root is unexcelled, but should *not* be employed if the stomach is in an irritated condition. Bitter Root is best when combined with other less harsh agents:

Tincture of Bitter Root (*Apocynum Androsaemifolium*)   5 to 10 drops
Tincture of Goldenseal (*Hydrastis canadensis*)   7 to 10 drops
Tincture of Fringe Tree (*Chiolanthus virginica*)   3 to 7 drops

In water between meals.

Dosage: *Tincture Apocynum* alone—5 to 10 drops in water before meals.

In small doses, Bitter Root is a laxative. As a tonic, 2 to 10 drops of the tincture before meals will stimulate the digestive organism. Bitter Root is an alterative in rheumatism, but is best combined with other agents for that purpose.

For emesis, 10 to 30 drops repeated every 30 minutes as necessary with plenty of water between doses.

Not as valuable as *Lobelia Inflata* for emesis.

BITTERSWEET

Solanum dulcamara

Common names: Woody Nightshade, Felonwort, Fever Twig, Violet Bloom, Scarlet Berry.

Generally known as the glandular, lymphatics medicine.

Bittersweet belongs in the old family domestic medicine chest, but is as effective today as it was when used only in infusion (when properly used), in glandular diseases and is especially soothing in irritable conditions. It is generally given in the form of syrup made with infusions, but is more certain when the tincture is used in conjunction with Queen's Root and various other alternatives. It has been found to be highly beneficial in the treatment of eczema, scrofula, and syphilis:

Tincture of Bittersweet (*Solanum dulcamara*)	10 to 15 drops
Tincture of Queen's Root (*Stillingia sylvatica*)	10 to 20 drops

In water 3 to 4 times a day.

Solanum is a mild narcotic and, for extreme nervousness and insomnia due to febrile conditions, it is best combined with *Passiflora:*

Tincture of Bittersweet (*Solanum dulcamara*)	10 to 20 drops
Tincture of Passion Flower (*Passiflora incarnata*)	15 to 30 drops

In water between meals and on retiring.

Bittersweet ointment is soothing and healing to irritable skin affections, piles, burns, scalds, and ulcers. Ointment is made by boiling 1 pound of the green crushed bark in 1 pound of lard or vase-

line. The home folks desire lard instead of vaseline, believing lard
to be more effective.

Dosage: Tincture *Solanum* alone, 10 to 20 drops in water 3 or 4
times a day.

Specifically: Solanum is a glandular, lymphatic agent and of
much service in skin and blood diseases.

The infusion, long a household or domestic medicine, is made
by boiling a tablespoonful of the cut or powdered root in a pint of
water for a few minutes and let steep one-half hour, 2 tablespoons
4 times a day.

BLACK COHOSH

Cimicifuga racemosa

Common names: Black Snakeroot, Rattlesnake Root, and Squaw
Root. It must *not* be confused with Squaw Vine, though like Squaw
Vine, it was an Indian remedy.

Black Cohosh is a relaxing nervine and expectorant. It acts
directly on the spinal nerve, and because of this action has been
much used with success in the treatment of St. Vitus dance and
spinal meningitis. So potent is the action of *Cimicifuga* that too
large doses of it may produce a dizzy feeling in the head, though it is
in no sense poisonous.

The Indian women depended almost wholly on it to relieve pain
during the menstrual period, and its use for this purpose has continued even among the general medical profession who still follow
a *natura* system of practice.

Cimicifuga is slightly narcotic; a sedative and an antispasmodic.

Due to its potency in relieving pain, *Cimicifuga* is frequently
combined with other agents for sciatica and rheumatism.

Dosage of the tincture of *Cimicifuga* alone, 10 to 20 drops when
and as indicated.

Cimicifuga is specifically a woman's remedy. Indicated in ovarian
neuralgia, rheumatic dysmenorrhea, and convulsions as a result of
nervous excitement, feeling of heavy weight in the sacral and lumbar

region, and hysterical spasms before or during menstrual period, melancholia and deep feeling of depression; dull aching headache. Best given in conjunction with *Pulsatilla*. SMALL frequent doses.

BLACK WILLOW
Salix nigra

Common names: Pussy Willow, Calkins Willow.
The woman's remedy:
Salix is an astringent and antiseptic and of much value in inflamed, ulcerated surfaces, hence indicated as a douche in viginitis, leucorrhea, and proctitis, for which either the infusion or tincture in warm water may be used.

Salix is a sedative in eroticism due to genito-urinary irritations such as prostatis, urethritis, and clitoric adhesions.

In domestic medicine it was and is used as a remedy for rheumatoid disorders and in inflamed joints, muscles, and nerves.

Dosage of tincture *Salix Nigra* alone, 10 to 20 drops according to symptoms.

Black Willow may be used as an infusion, but the tincture or fluid extracts are more certain in their action.

BLUEBERRY
Vaccinium Myrtillus

Other names: Bilberry, Whortle Berry, Burren Myrtle, Huckleberry.

Although Blueberry and NOT Huckleberry leaves have been a folk remedy in many parts of the world (from Pennsylvania to the Austrian Alps) in the treatment of the control of diabetes, the medical profession generally did not admit that it contained any ingredient or active principle of value in diabetes.

It was not until an Austrian physician, Dr. R. U. Wagner came to America, and in association with Dr. Frederick M. Allen at the Psychiatric Institution of Morristown, New Jersey, reported in *Collier's,* March 17, 1928, and engaged in serious experimentation and research and discovered an active principle with a "remarkable potency to reduce excess sugar in the blood" which they named Mythillin.

These physicians found that, though this acted slowly, it was wholly harmless even in excessive amounts, generally efficient, though it could not replace insulin in chronic cases.

The results of these experiments, and cases treated with good results according to the *National Weekly* were reported before the American Medical Association and in the *Journal* of the American Medical Association.

While the leaves of Huckleberry may be used, the Blueberry leaves *are to be preferred by far*. An infusion—always freshly made —by the infusion of a teaspoon of the leaves in a cup of boiling water, for one-half an hour and taken two to three times a day.

Many, so afflicted, combine Strawberry leaves and Thyme (*Thymus Vulgaris*) with *Myrtillus,* one teaspoonful of each in 8 ounces of boiling water, dividing into three portions, one portion each forenoon, afternoon, and evening.

Dosage of tincture *Myrtillus* alone, 15 to 40 drops in water 3 or more times a day. The infusion is to be preferred in domestic use.

BLUE FLAG

Iris versicolor

Common names: Flag Lily, Liver Lily, Water Flag, Snake Lily.

Called the lymphatic and thyroid gland remedy. It is indicated in most non-malignant enlargements.

Natural agents for this purpose are few—among them more especially iodine and foods containing it, kelp and thyroid. This is a valuable and welcome addition.

It is also clearly indicated in hepatic conditions, when due to the ingestions of congesting foods causing constipation and indigestion, headache, and dizziness.

It is one of the very few remedies that has any influence in correcting milk-colored, clay-colored stools in adults.

Dosage of tincture alone, 10 to 25 drops in water, 3 times a day.

BONESET

Eupatorium perfoliatum

Common names: Thoroughwort, Indian Sage, Ague Weed.

Eupatorium is largely of the nature of *Asclepias,* but is harsher and more powerful in its action. It should be used in place, or in conjunction with, *Asclepias* to combat miasmatic and malarial influences. It is especially indicated in fevers, where there is aching of the bones.

The cold infusion or tincture is a tonic and aperient. The warm infusion is diaphoretic and when given in too large an amount is emetic, for which *Lobelia* is superior.

As a tonic it is useful in remittent, intermittent and typhoid fevers, dyspepsia, and general debility. In intermittent fever a strong infusion, as hot as can be comfortably swallowed, or the tincture in hot water, is to be administered for the purpose of emesis, if *Lobelia* is not procurable.

During the intermission, the cold infusion, or tincture, in cold water is given every hour as a tonic and antiperiodic. In epidemic influences (la grippe) the warm infusion is of much value as an emetic and diaphoretic, likewise in febrile diseases such as catarrh, colds, and like attacks.

For influenza or the grippe, give:

Tincture of Boneset (*Eupatorium perfoliatum*)	15 to 30 drops
Tincture of Pleurisy Root (*Asclepias tuberosa*)	20 to 40 drops
Tincture of Skullcap (*Scutellaria Lateriflora*)	12 to 15 drops

In hot water every 1, 2, or 3 hours. It is well to immediately cleanse the stomach by emetics at the onset of the disease, and then give only sufficient of the above to control the chills, and produce a cleansing perspiration. Where chills are extreme, *Capsicum,* in 2-, 4-, or 5-grain doses may be given with this preparation. Hardly a case need be lost by death, and there are no aftereffects of the disease.

Tincture of *Cinchona,* Peruvian Bark: 10 to 30 drops may be added to this formula in severe cases, where there is much pain.

Infusions of *Eupatorium,* given hot and in fairly large doses, is an active agent, producing copious diaphoresis, and in the treatment of catarrhal colds and acute malarial fevers, is productive of much good. It has always been a domestic remedy, formerly familiar to mothers in districts where medical aid was not easily obtainable.

It is part of the *Natura* physician's armamentarium.

Dosage tincture of *Eupatorium* alone, 15 to 40 drops as indicated by age and condition.

Infusion: One teaspoon of the powdered herb; steep in a cup of boiling water for half an hour. One teaspoon every 3 hours. More or less frequently, and either in hot or cold water, according to condition.

Eupatorium may be combined with the various agents as indicated by *Asclepias*.

Eupatorium is invaluable in the treatment of every type of illness, where there is a temperature and aching of the bones.

Specifically: intermittent fever, "la grippe," especially where there is soreness of the bones and muscles, catarrhal, and bilious fever accompanied by thirst for cold water causing vomiting and lack of perspiration. In coryza with sneezing, a long used, valuable agent. Combines well with *Geranium Maculatum,* Cranesbill.

BUCHU

Barosma betulina

Common name: Bookoo.

Best known as a gravel and chronic prostatis remedy.

Barosma is an aromatic and a stimulant, a diuretic, and a diaphoretic. It is frequently prescribed in chronic inflammation of the bladder, irritation of the membrane of the urethra, uric-acid gravel, diabetes in its first stages, and incontinence of the urine. It is of benefit in chronic prostatis.

Dose of the tincture, 10 to 60 drops.

It is best when combined with the more active remedies indicated in the conditions mentioned.

Buchu, because of its mild action, was formerly a much used household remedy in the form of infusion: one teaspoonful of the herb to the cup of boiling water, steep half an hour. Drink when cold. Two cups a day, or more often when indicated.

Dosage of tincture of *Barosma* 10 to 20 drops in water, 3 times a day.

BURDOCK
Arctium Lappa—Lappa Major

Common names: Clot-bur, Bardana, Lappa.

The root and seed of *Lappa Articum* is a soothing demulcent tonic alternative. It slowly, but steadily, influences the skin, soothes the kidneys, and relieves the lymphatics. It is of great value in the treatment of all skin diseases and in scrofulous affections. It is soothing to the mucous membrane throughout the entire system, hence is valuable in irritated conditions. Its soothing character is also extended to the serous membrane and is valuable in rheumatism especially if combined with more stimulating agents like *Hydrastis* and *Barosma Crenata:*

Tincture of Burdock Root (*Arctium Lappa*)	10 to 20 drops
Tincture of Goldenseal (*Hydrastis canadensis*)	8 to 12 drops
Tincture of Buchu (*Barosma betulina*)	10 to 15 drops

In water, 3 to 4 times a day.

The infusion or tincture in hot water influences the sebaceous glands and is of importance in scarlatina, other exanthema, and also in typhoid fever. In all these conditions it should be combined with coneflower.

Tincture of Burdock Root (*Arctium Lappa*)	10 to 20 drops
Tincture of Coneflower (*Echinacea Angustifolia*)	20 to 40 drops

In warm water as frequently as indicated by the symptoms. Moisture of the skin must be controlled by the addition of tincture of scullcap 2 to 5 drops.

When this formula is used in the treatment of typhoid fever, tincture of wild indigo, 2 to 5 drops.

In domestic practice, an infusion is made with 1 teaspoon of the powdered root to a cup of boiling water, steep one half hour, strain. One to 2 cups a day.

Dosage of the tincture of Burdock alone, 10 to 25 drops in water, 3 to 4 times a day.

CACTUS
Cereus grandiflorus

Common name: Night-blooming Cereus.
General indications: Cardiac disorders of an inorganic nature.

Feeling of constriction of the heart as from iron bands. Feeling of heart weakness. Heart action rapid, short, irregular with possible great difficulty in breathing, or chronic slow action.

The dominant effect of *Cactus* is that of an antispasmodic upon the heart in a chronic condition. It is indicated in angina, or pseudo-anginal conditions, cardiac spasms, spasmodic asthma, and wherever the heart muscles are concerned. It cannot substitute for digitalis or glonoin in acute heart attacks.

Dosage: Two to 10 drops, 3 or 4 times a day. It is best combined with *Crataegus oxyacantha.*

Specifically: *Cactus Grandiflora* is indicated by a frequent feeling of constrictions of the heart where there is no organic condition. Short, rapid, irregular heart beat. Acute pain or "stitches" in the heart. Difficulty in breathing. It is a dependable non-toxic heart remedy.

CHAMOMILE, COMMON

Anthemis nobilis

Common names: Chamomilla; German, Chamomile; Camomile.

In general use *Chamomile* has maintained a well-earned reputation for unknown number of years, and its usefulness is as fully recognized by the *Natura* physicians as it has been in family use.

In action it is a soothing nervine and a mild stomach tonic to be given where there is weakness and poor appetite and the *tendency to melancholy.*

In some respects it has been called a "children's remedy," of much use in light fevers, restlessness in children, and to make certain that in such ailments as measles and other children's illnesses, the usual rash is not retarded. In all such ailments the infusion is of greatest service. A tablespoon of the herb in a half pint of hot water and steeped for half an hour. Dosage: One teaspoon every half hour for results. For this purpose the common garden variety, therefore called an "old woman's" remedy, is most desirable, though both the Roman and German varieties are good.

When given in the warm infusion, a teaspoon to part of a cup of warm water, *Chamomile* will promote perspiration, so desirable in most cases of fevers, and may be given in connection with almost every other herbal medication. In women, it helps promote the menstrual flow, though the tincture in hot water will serve the same purpose. The cold infusion is a tonic and suitable in stomach difficulties in conjunction with other agents. It serves well as a drink during convalescence from febrile diseases. Before the advent of fruit juices, it was the standard liquid drink in practically all diseases where a temperature was present. It serves just as well now.

In extreme nervous conditions, where the stomach is at fault, best results are obtained by making use of the formula:

Tincture of Chamomile (*Anthemis nobilis*)	10 to 20 drops
Tincture of Valerian	10 to 20 drops

In water every three hours or as indicated according to age and symptoms. Always best given in warm liquids.

In doses of from 5 to 10 drops of the tincture, it relieves the nervous irritation and false pains of the later months of gestation. Equal part of *Squaw Vine* may be combined with it. It is also of great value in cases of nervous dyspepsia and sick headache during the menstrual period and is well adapted as a mild antispasmodic to neurotic women. Motherwort combines well with it.

Anthemis may be classed as a stimulant, tonic, and antispasmodic. It is especially useful as a child's remedy, being of much service in flatulent colic so frequently met with in small infants.

"Atony of the entire system is another reason for employing this agent, its action being more pronounced in cases of atony or debility of any parts of the digestive apparatus.

"Wrongs of the menstrual functions, caused by debility, are frequently righted by the use of this medication. Atony is the key to its specific action." *Dr. Gowes—Lloyd.*

Anthemis, in combination with hops, made into a poultice will relieve sprains, bruises, and swellings and also help to restore shrunken sinews. *Lobelia* combines well with it:

Tincture of Chamomile (*Anthemis nobilis*)	15 to 30 drops
Tincture of Indian Tobacco (*Lobelia inflata*)	3 to 9 drops
Tincture of Hops (*Humulus Lupulus*)	20 to 40 drops

Apply warm, change every few hours.

Specifically: Matricaria has long been a household or domestic remedy for many uses and is a dependable agent. It is a nervine, stimulant and dipthoretic, hence its manifold indications. It is of much value in functional disorders in both children and women. During dentition it reduces nervousness, irritability, and emotional manifestations, as well as restlessness and sleeplessness. It is equally valuable in flatulence and colic during this period. In the beginning of colds, in combination with *Asclepias,* Pleurisy Root, it is of utmost value. In these conditions, it is best given as an infusion.

It has long been used by women during premenstrual and menstrual periods to relieve dysmenorrhic spasms, and promotes the menses when due to exposure to colds, uterine spasms or nervous tension.

Matricaria is indicated and dependable in neurotic and emotional manifestations, muscular twitchings, general uneasiness, and sleeplessness. In all of these manifestations, it may be taken in infusion or tincture and combines well for other agents for the same purposes.

Externally, it frequently relieves or eliminates eczema when applied in an infusion, alone or combined with Calendula, Marigold. It is indispensable in the *Armamentarium* of the *Natura* physician.

Dosage of tincture *Anthemis* alone, 10 to 20 drops in water, 3 to 4 times a day.

CLIVERS

Galium aparine

Common names: Cleaverswort, Bed Straw, Catchweed, Goosegrass, Cleavers.

A diaphoretic in fevers where a free outward circulation should be quickly established. It is a highly valuable refrigerant and diuretic, and beneficial in suppression of the urine, calculous affections, inflammation of the kidneys and bladder, and in the scalding of urine in gonorrhoea.

During certain stages of scarlet fever and like infections where there is a tendency to irritable conditions of the kidneys, Clivers will prove highly beneficial as a tea or tincture in which other more active agents may be given. For children and adults who suffer from scalding urine, it is *the* remedy. In the inflammatory stages of gonorrhoea, it will relieve the irritation and sooth the nervous system.

Indicated in all conditions where the mucous membrane in any part of the system, is in an irritated condition:

Tincture of Clivers (*Galium aparine*)   20 to 30 drops
Tincture of Buchu (*Barosma betulina*)   10 to 12 drops
In water 3 or 4 times a day.

Dosage: Tincture of *Clivers* alone, 20 to 30 drops in water as indicated.

CONEFLOWER

Echinacea angustifolia

Common names: Wild Niggerhead; Purple Cone Flower; Black Sampson; Kansas Niggerhead; Brauneria pallida; Rudbeckia pallida.

Thomsonian, Physio-Medical and *Natura* physicians have always maintained that *Echinacea* is a herbal, natural antitoxin. Orthodox physicians have not generally been willing to accept it as such, though many do. It is a controversial agent.

"*Echinacea* is a corrector of the deprivations of the body fluids," was Dr. Niederkorn's opinion, and this, whether the morbific changes of the fluids of the body are internal, or caused by external introductions. Its use is indicated in septic infections, septicemia in its various forms, blood poisoning, adynamic fevers, typhoid fever, cellular abscesses, salpingitis, carbuncles, cancerous cachexia, and in fevers or conditions where there is a bluish discoloration of the mucous membranes, tongue brownish or almost black, or when discharges are foul—in fact, in any or all conditions which point to sepsis.

Discriminating physicians of all schools have found it invaluable in infections, both internal and external, strumous conditions (where an alternative is indicated), peritonitis, acute fevers, syphilitic conditions, puerperal infection, infections with tendency to abscess, bites and stings of poisonous insects and reptiles, typhoid infections, blood perversions, toxemia with and without fever, septicemia, erysipelas, acute infections, gangrenous conditions, diptheria, or wherever there is a formation of pus suppurations as in tonsilitis, infected sores, and wounds.

CORN SILK

Stigmata Maydis

Common name: Indian Corn—the silk.

Stigmata Maidis possesses great virtue in irritated conditions of the urinary organs and is believed to be the only known remedy capable of cleansing the kidneys from the dangerous deposits of brick dust in the urine and removing the condition which is the cause of it. Frequently referred to as the brick dust remover.

"*Stigmata Maidis* is indicated in cystic irritation, due to phosphatic and uric acid concretions. In these cases the urine is usually scant and of a strong odor. The remedy not only relieves the bladder and urethral irritation, but tends also to prevent the formation of gravel and calculi. It is an important and favorite remedy in the treatment of urinal disorders of the aged, especially where the urine is strong and scant, and shows a heavy sediment. *Stigmata* should always be thought of in inflammatory conditions of the urethra, bladder, and kidneys, where it is evident that the inflammatory trouble is due to the presence of urinary concretions."—*Dr. Neiderkorn—Lloyd.*

Where there is a tendency to the formation of gravel, or where it is known to exist, give:

Tincture of Corn Silk (*Stigmata Maydis*)	10 to 20 drops
Tincture of Couch-Grass (*Triticum repens*)	5 to 15 drops

In water as required. Dose of *Stigmata Maidis* alone, 10 to 60 drops.

As a domestic remedy, a syrup is made of 4 ounces of Corn Silk, and one-half pound of Dandelion root. Steep in quart of boiling water half an hour, then add 2 ounces Goldenseal. Dose, 1 teaspoonful in half cup of water, every 3 or 4 hours or as needed for relief.

For bedwetting:

Tincture of Corn Silk (*Stigmata maydis*)	15 to 30 drops
Tincture of Agrimony (*Agrimonia Eupatoria*)	10 to 30 drops

In water between meals and bedtime.

Dosage: Tincture of *Stigmata Maidis* 15 to 30 drops in water, 3 or 4 times a day.

Stigmata Maidis is indicated in practically all formulae for urinary disorders.

COUCH-GRASS

Triticum or *Agropyron repens*

Common names: Quick-Grass, Dog-Grass, Durfa Grass.

Called the kidney, bladder and gravel remedy. One of the old domestic remedies.

Medically, *Triticum* is classed as a mild, stimulating demulcent acting chiefly upon the kidneys, bladder, and urethra, and is especially valuable in gravel, many experienced physicians claiming that its timely use has dissolved small calculi. It is indicated by catarrhal and purulent discharges from the urethra, in purulent cystitis, incipient nephritis, stangury, enlarged prostate (when due to chronic gonorrhoea), gout, jaundice, and rheumatism. In incontinence of the urine with intense burning sensation and constant desire to urinate, it is splendid in its results. Dose 5 to 30 drops. To help calculi to pass, the maximum dose of 40 to 60 drops in hot water should be given.

In chronic gonorrhoea:

Tincture of Couch-Grass (*Triticum repens*)	5 to 20 drops
Tincture of Goldenseal (*Hydrastis canadensis*)	7 to 10 drops
Tincture of Sandalwood (*Santalum album*)	10 to 20 drops
Tincture of Buchu (*Barosma betulina*)	10 to 20 drops

Dosage: In water three or more times a day.

For enlarged prostate (non-operative):

Tincture of Couch-Grass (*Triticum repens*)	5 to 15 drops
Tincture of Fringe Tree (*Chiolanthus virginica*)	3 to 7 drops
Tincture of Saw Palmetto (*Sarenoa serrulata*)	5 to 20 drops

In water, three or four times a day.

In rheumatism complicated with prostatic involvement:

Tincture of Couch-Grass (*Triticum repens*)	5 to 20 drops
Tincture of Motherwort (*Leonurus cardiaca*)	9 to 15 drops
Tincture of Scurvy Grass (*Cochlearia officinalis*)	7 to 15 drops
Tincture of Black Cohosh (*Cimicifuga racemosa*)	1 to 15 drops

In water, three or four times a day. *Black Cohosh* should be used with caution.

Dosage: Tincture of *Couch-Grass* alone, 10 to 20 drops in water, 2 or more times a day.

Specifically: One of the most important symptoms for the prescribing of *Triticum* is a burning sensation and constant desire to urinate.

CROWFOOT

Geranium Maculatum

Common names: Dove's-Foot, Crowfoot, Wild Alum Root, Spotted Geranium, Wild Geranium, Cranesbill.

Caution. It is not to be confused with *Ranunculus Bulbosus,* also of the Crowfoot family and undesirable as a medical agent.

The root is a pleasant, positive tonic astringent. It is only moderately drying, but is persistent and effective—one of the most potent and excellent astringent agents. Its chief influence is upon the alvine mucous membranes. It is applicable in the treatment of a sore mouth or gums, mercurial salivation, spongy gums, catarrhal ophthalmia, leukorrhoea, gleet, dystentery, and diarrhea.

It is a splendid and dependable local and constitutional styptic for hemorrhages from the nose, lungs, stomach, bowels, or uterus, and for this purpose is best combined with Bayberry:

Tincture of Cranesbill (*Geranium Maculatum*)	10 to 30 drops
Tincture of Bayberry (*Myrica Cerifera*)	13 to 30 drops
Tincture of Myrrh (*Commiphora myrrha*)	2 to 4 drops

In typhoid fever where there is excessive discharge, whether fecal or canious, this agent is one of the most valuable. In this condition it should be combined:

Tincture of Cranesbill (*Geranium Maculatum*)	10 to 30 drops
Tincture of Coneflower (*Echinacea angustifolia*)	10 to 30 drops

In water according to symptoms, or it may be combined with:

Tincture of Cranesbill (*Geranium Maculatum*)	10 to 30 drops
Tincture of Wild Indigo (*Baptisia tinctoria*)	2 to 15 drops

Dosage: In water every 3 or 4 hours.

In emergencies, where the tinctures cannot be had, 2 teaspoons of Cranesbill, *Geranium* and one teaspoon of *Baptisia,* wild indigo, ground roots may be steeped in a cup of hot water for 30 minutes; then give 1 teaspoon of the infusion every 2 or 3 hours.

There are few agents which possess a wider range of usefulness than *Geranium Maculatum,* and which are so devoid of harmful properties. In all forms of hemorrhage, whether internal or external, hemoptysis usually can be arrested promptly by 30 to 50 doses of the tincture, given hourly until controlled. Relapse may be prevented by continuing the same dose at longer intervals for three or four days. In hemorrhage from the kidneys and the intestinal canal, better results will be obtained by the administration of smaller doses, 20 drops four times a day, for an extended period. This is the only practical way of using it in chronic cases. Epistaxis may be checked speedily by plugging the nostrils with cotton dipped in a solution composed of one part each of the tincture of *Geranium* and *Bayberry* combined with vaginal injections of the same combination.

In hemorrhage of the stomach, 30 to 50 drops will often relieve when all other agents have failed.

Where there is pain and distress from gastric ulcers, *Geranium* will relieve, and in many instances cure the trouble. In cases of pulmonary hemorrhages, it is the remedy in doses of 40 to 50 drops of the tincture; after its action has been established, it may be given in doses of 10 to 15 drops, three or four times a day to guard against the hemorrhages returning.

In consumption it will modify the night-sweats and cough, and control the diarrhea that is so annoying and always weakening to the patient.

In the treatment of chronic bronchitis by its action in condensing the relaxed bronchial membrane, we check the cough and profuse expectoration, and thereby strengthen the patient.

"In the weakened stomach of hard drinkers we find an admirable place for *Geranium.* In such cases, *Capsicum,* 3 drops, should be added to each dose. Chronic gonorrhoea and gleet are cured by the local injection of a 10 to 25 per cent solution. It is valuable in the treatment of sore mouth, either mercurial or from other cause. Use diluted as a wash and give internally. In the treatment of leukorrhoea where there is a relaxed and atonic condition, make a tampon of surgical wool, and after saturating with the full-strength extract, push well up against the uterus. In uterine catarrh and relaxed conditions it is a splendid remedy. In prolapsus of the bowels, wet the protruding parts with the strong non-alcoholic fluid and inject

25 per cent solution into the bowels three or four times a week. The same treatment will cure many cases of recent hemorrhoids. It is excellent for nasal polypi by injecting them with the tincture. The polypoid growth will degenerate and drop out after a time—*Drs. Comfort and Lyle.*

In all hemorrhages, whether from nose, throat, lungs, kidneys, bowels, or uterine:

Tincture of Cranesbill (*Geranium Maculatum*)	10 to 30 drops
Tincture of Bayberry (*Myrica cerifera*)	15 to 30 drops

In water every hour or 2 as indicated by symptoms.

Dosage of the tincture *Geranium* alone, 10 to 30 drops in water every hour or two, indicated by age and condition.

Specifically: "*Geranium* is a powerful non-irritating astringent, to the relief of conditions exhibiting relaxed, atonic, and enfeebled tissues with copious, debilitating discharges. It is of value in chronic diarrhea with mucus discharges, chronic dysentery, menorrhagia, diarrhea of subacute character with constant desire to evacuate the bowels. Passive forms of hemorrhage often are controlled by it as it exerts a good influence in hemantinuria and is of considerable value in catarrhal gastritis. Should be employed during the *active* stages of inflammation." *Dr. King—Lloyd.*

DOGWOOD, AMERICAN

Cornus Florida

Common names: Boxwood, Flowering Cornet, Green Ozier.

Cornus contains an active principle Cornine, a splendid substitute for *Cinchona,* Peruvian Bark or Quinine, and used for the same purpose. It is free from the effects of Quinine when continued for too long a period—after chills are controlled.

Dosage: Tincture *Cornus* alone, 20 to 40 drops in water according to symptoms.

It is an old family remedy used in place of *Cinchona* or *Quinine* and is made into an infusion: One teaspoonful steeped in a cup of boiling water for half an hour; one-half cup three times a day, or as required.

DOGWOOD, JAMAICA

Piscidia erythrina

The Natura physician's agent as a substitute for narcotics, generally prescribed in nervous, neurotic conditions. *Piscidia becomes toxic in overdoses.*

Piscidia's place in natural medication is to counteract nervousness and insomnia due to some form of hysterian and nervous tension.

It is of value in facial and sciatic neuralgia.

It gives excellent service in dysmenorrhea when accompanied with cramps, nervousness, and sleeplessness, but is most effective when combined with *Black Haw:*

Tincture of Jamaica Dogwood (*Piscidia erythrina*)	1 to 20 drops
Tincture of Black Haw (*Viburnum opulus*)	5 to 15 drops

In hot water as frequently as necessary.

ELECAMPANE

Inula Helenium

Common names: Elf Dock, Scabwort, Velvet Dock.

Generally known as the anti-tuberculin remedy, although there is no proof that it is of much benefit in the treatment of the disorders which indicate the onset of consumption, it may not actually deserve the name of an anti-tuberculin agent, despite the fact that there was much faith in it as a household remedy.

It is a compound agent; an expectorant, an excellent tonic, and cough remedy, a stomachic, and a diuretic.

Elecampane is important in the treatment of general catarrhal conditions, controls mucous discharges, and as a tonic it encourages metabolism; hence its value in incipient tuberculosis.

Best given in fluid extract, 20 to 40 drops, three or more times a day.

EVENING PRIMROSE

Oenothera biennis

Common name: Tree primrose.

This is not to be confused with Butter Rose *(Primula veris).*

This agent is indicated in neurotic—mental depression—conditions resulting in the development of alimentary toxins due to a long continued faulty diet creating toxic waste which causes depression of the solar plexus—the nerve center.

Evening Primrose stimulates digestion by vitalizing the stomach and has a direct influence on the liver and spleen. It should be combined with other agents for the purpose of eliminating the toxic waste. According to symptoms, bile salts should generally be prescribed in conjunction with it.

Dosage of tincture of Evening Primrose alone, 5 to 40 drops according to symptoms.

An authority, Dr. Unruh, speaking of *Echinacea,* states:

"The drug is found to produce direct stimulation of the katabolic processes, increase in the flow of saliva, sweat, and urine, and increase in glandular activity. It thus *antagonizes all septic processes, facilitates the elimination of toxins from the organism, and lastly, it has a destructive effect upon the streptococci, staphylococci, and other pyogenic organisms.*"

This has always been, and still is, the opinion of the modern *Natura* physician based on experience.

There is no morbid condition in which *Echinacea* is not indicated, and its greatest benefit has been manifest in typhoid fever.

When there is extreme morbidity, Myrrh should be combined with it:

Tincture of Myrrh (*Commiphora myrrha*)	2 to 5 drops
Tincture of Coneflower (*Echinacea angustifolia*)	15 to 30 drops

Every 1 to 3 hours, according to the condition. When *Echinacea* is applied externally to neutralize morbid conditions or insect bites, Myrrh, equal parts, should always be combined with it.

Dosage of tincture *Echinacea alone,* 15 to 30 drops in water every 1 to 3 hours as indicated. The action of *Echinacea,* is like antitoxin in various types of blood poisoning, infections of different nature, and causes in the most morbid conditions.

Specifically: *Echinacea* is the *Natura* physician's antitoxin.

FEVERFEW

Chrysanthemum Parthenium

Common names: Featherfew, Febrifuge Plant, Batchelor's Buttons.

In hot infusions or the tincture in hot water, it is a diaphoretic and relieves the head, brain, and nerves from pressure and excitement. In pleuritis, it relieves the hyperemia present, and reduces the inflammatory excitement. During parturition by equalizing the circulation, the pains become more regular, the contractions firmer, and the rigid *os uteri* relieved of its tensity. In cases where the menses are suppressed due to cold, it quickly relieves the hyperemia present, and the flow assumes its normal condition.

The influence of Feverfew upon the circulation tends toward the surface, and with proper hepatics it assists in relieving the circulation of impurities, especially in uremia and cholemia. It is a superior tonic to the stomach relieving hyperemic conditions of the mucous membrane and is serviceable in colic, flatulence, eructions, and general indigestion.

In bronchitis and pneumonia, it dispels hyperemia and tones the mucous membranes when combined with *Asclepias:*

Tincture of Pleurisy Root (*Asclepias tuberose*)	10 to 20 drops
Tincture of Feverfew (*Chrysanthemum Parthenium*)	10 to 20 drops

In puerperal fever, it is an important agent when combined with Echinacea:

Tincture of Feverfew (*Chrysanthemum Parthenium*)	10 to 30 drops
Tincture of Coneflower (*Echinacea angustifolia*)	10 to 20 drops
Tincture of Cayenne Pepper (*Capsicum frutescens*) (*Capsicum minimum*)	2 to 3 drops

Every 2 to 3 hours depending on symptoms.

Dosage of the tincture *Chrysanthemum* alone, 10 to 30 drops in water every 2 or 3 hours, as indicated by condition.

In nervous unstrung conditions as a result of toxic effects of too great indulgence in alcoholic beverages, 15 to 40 drops of the tincture, as often as required, usually give good results.

In domestic use, a teaspoon of the herb is steeped in a cup of boiling water half an hour, 1 or 2 cups a day in tablespoon doses.

In hot compresses Feverfew may be applied with benefit over the lungs, stomach or abdomen in either congestions or inflammation.

Specifically : *Chrysanthemum* is a dependable tonic, carminative, and stimulant. It is diffusive, mildly stimulating, and a relaxing agent. It influences the skin, nervous system, the circulation, and the genito-urinary organism.

FRINGE TREE

Chionanthus virginica

Common name : Poison ash, sometimes called Old Man's Beard.

"*Chionanthus* exerts a special influence upon the liver, and to a slight extent upon all the organs engaged in digestion and blood-making. The indication for its exhibition are : yellowness of the skin and eyes ; slight or fully-developed jaundice with a sense of uneasiness and general pain simulating colic. It is one of the most certain remedies employed, whether the case is one of jaundice, formation and passage of gallstone, bilious colic (indicated by yellowness of skin), acute dyspepsia, acute or chronic inflammation of the liver, or the irritable liver of the hard drinker.

"*Chionanthus* is also indicated by a dirty, sallow skin, with expressionless eyes and hepatic tenderness ; the passage of light grayish stools and scant urine which stains the clothing yellow. The liver-pain of *Chionanthus* may range from a slight uneasiness with a feeling of weight and fullness to an intense pain converging from the gall-bladder to the umbilicus and attended with nausea, vomiting, and marked prostration." *Dr. Felter—Lloyd.*

The dosage of the tincture is from 5 to 10 drops in water.

Whenever there is jaundice or other affliction during pregnancy which indicates that the liver is not functioning normally, *Chionanthus* in 5 to 10 drops in water before meals is indicated.

In malignant tumors of the stomach or bowels and in uterine tumors, a combination of :

Tincture of Goldenseal (*Hydrastis canadensis*)	7 to 10 drops
Tincture of Fringe Tree (*Chiolanthus virginica*)	3 to 7 drops

Dose 10 to 20 drops in water before meals and at bedtime has proven effective.

This same formula is indicated in most chronic conditions of the liver where symptoms indicate the spleen may be affected.

In bilious colic it is best first to cleanse the stomach by giving an emetic dose of Lobelia and when this is accomplished, follow with:

Tincture of Fringe Tree (*Chiolanthus virginica*)	4 to 7 drops
Tincture of Goldenseal (*Hydrastis canadensis*)	7 to 10 drops

It has been generally believed that the medical properties of *Chionanthus* cannot be extracted by infusions, though it has long been used as a family medicine by steeping the cut bark and root in hot water for half an hour and this divided throughout the day.

The powdered root and bark has been widely used in the treatment of wounds and irritations that do not readily yield to usual treatment. May be combined with other healing agents.

The Physio-Medical and *Natura* physicians in general practice would not think of treating liver and spleen conditions without this agent.

Dosage: Tincture *Chionanthus* alone, 7 to 10 drops in water according to indication.

Specifically: *Chionanthus Virginica* is *the spleen remedy*. It is indicated in congestions of the liver, especially where constipation is present, and the possibility of formation of gall-stones, jaundice, and conditions arising as a result of splenic inaction. Best when combined with *Hydrastis,* goldenseal.

GENTIAN, YELLOW

Genitiana lutea

Common names: Gentian Lutea.

The tincture generally used in medical practice is prepared from the imported herb. It is mild, but a decidedly bitter tonic.

Its chief action is upon the liver and stomach. For sluggishness of the liver with general dyspepsia, it is of great value. For ague it will often prove effective when other agents fail, but should be combined with *Capsicum* and *Lobelia*:

Tincture of Gentian (*Georgiana lutea*)	3 to 10 drops
Tincture of Indian Tobacco (*Lobelia inflata*)	3 to 10 drops
Tincture of Cayenne Pepper (*Capsicum frutescens*)	
(*Capsicum minimum*)	1 to 3 drops

This should be repeated every hour. For chills give only in hot water.

"Gentian is one of the most popular of the simple (non-poisonous) bitter tonics, and as such finds its best field in atonic states of the gastro-intestinal tract with feeble or slow digestion. It improves the appetite, increases digestion, augments the circulation, and tends to raise the heat of the body. In small doses it is valuable to relieve irritation, and improve the appetite and the digestion after protracted fevers when vitality is low. An indication for gentian is: Depressed feeling in the pit of the stomach and a sense of physical and mental weariness."—*Dr. Scudder—Lloyd.*

Tincture of Yellow Gentian (*Gentiana lutea*)	3 to 10 drops
Tincture of Goldenseal (*Hydrastis canadensis*)	8 to 12 drops
Tincture of Indian Tobacco (*Lobelia inflata*)	3 to 8 drops

In water 3 times a day, before meals.

There is an American Gentian, blue flowered and very common in many states, more especially in Pennsylvania. This is also one of those "old woman's" agents and frequently used in stomach conditions. Like many remedies common among the people, it is gathered when in bloom. Place approximately 2 ounces of the crushed flower tops and sometimes the roots also into a bottle with a pint of brandy or grain alcohol, allow to stand for a week shaking frequently, and it is ready for use. The dosage is from 1 teaspoonful to 1 tablespoonful in water, taken either before or after meals, and more frequently in acute conditions. The amount made usually depends on the size of the family and the number of those more or less afflicted with digestive disturbances.

Dosage of tincture *Gentiana* alone, 4 to 10 drops in water before meals.

GUM PLANT

Grindelia comporum
Grindelia cuneifolia
Grindelia squarrosa

Common name: Grindelia.
The ivy poison (rhus) and oak poisoning remedy. In nearly

60 years of practicing we have found no agent more effective in this, sometimes horrible affliction, than *Grindelia*.

Grindelia is equally indicated when applied to indolent ulcers, impetigo, eczema, and allergic dermatitis. The preparation of this remedy which has offered the best results is prepared by combining 1 ounce of fluid extract of Gum Plant, *Grindelia,* 1 ounce of 90 proof alcohol, and 1 or two ounces of water, and applied as frequently as the itch demands. At night a compress made with it may be applied to the affected portions of the body. In conjunction with the outward application, it should be given internally: Tincture of *Grindelia,* 5 to 20 drops in water according to age and conditions, 3 or 4 times a day.

Grindelia is also indicated in asthma, bronchial, or allergic cases, and respiratory conditions with which harsh, dry coughs and wheezing are associated. It is of no value to asthma where the heart is involved.

Dosage: Tincture of *Grindelia* alone, 5 to 30 drops according to age or condition.

HAWTHORN

Crataegus oxyacantha

Common name: Hawthorn Berries, May, May Blossom, Whitethorn.

Non-organic, irregular, and feeble heart action, vulvular murmurs. Dyspnea on least exertion, irregular pulse action. Hypertension. Not stimulative.

Mild cases of diminished heart reserve are conditions when the *Natura* physician seeks to avoid prescribing toxic drugs.

Crataegus, in combination with *Cactus grandiflorus,* is the ideal agent, being non-toxic it may be administered as long as necessary without ill effects.

"*Crataegus* is a mild and non-poisonous cardiac remedy with anti-spasmodic properties that render it a valuable drug in angina pectoris. It is to be considered more of a sedative and regulator of the heart than a stimulant."—*Dr. Thomas F. Reilly.*

Crataegus should not be given in large doses, as it may cause nausea:

Tincture of Hawthorn (*Crataegus oxyacantha*)   12 drops
Tincture of Cactus (*Cereus grandiflorus*)   2 drops

Dosage: Three or 4 times a day. The combination tablet is to be preferred to the tincture.

Specifically: The *Cactus* and *Crataegus* combination is a "sustaining" agent indicated in cardiac conditions when a frequent or constant toning effect is necessary. It is non-toxic or irritating to the digestive organism. It will not substitute where *Digitalis* or *Glonoin* is indicated.

HOREHOUND

Marrubium vulgare

Common name: Marrabium, Horehound.

Horehound is an old domestic remedy formerly employed in the family in the treatment of colds and coughs.

Medically it is classed as a stimulant, diaphoretic, and slightly laxative. In such cases it is given as a hot infusion or as a tincture in hot water. The hot infusion or tincture in hot water serves best when combined with other agents for the purpose intended.

The infusion or tincture given cold is a bitter tonic, useful in consumptive coughs. In syrup it is a tonic and expectorant.

"Horehound is an effective expectorant and stimulant in breaking up recent colds, bronchitis, bronchial catarrh, and certain types of asthma where there is mucous expectoration, dyspnea and aphonia, and laryngitis."—*Dr. Verbon.*

Horehound infusion, or tincture in hot water, sweetened with honey is excellent in asthma and all complaints of the lungs and bronchial tubes. The syrup made with honey and kept on hand in many families is used to loosen tough phlegm and harshness caused by colds.

In deep-seated colds with cough, it is best combined with *Asclepias* and *Scutellaria:*

Tincture of Scullcap (*Scutellaria Laterifolia*)   2 to 15 drops
Tincture of Pleurisy Root (*Asclepias tuberosa*)   20 to 45 drops
Tincture of Horehound (*Marrubium vulgara*)   5 to 40 drops

In warm water every 2 or 3 hours according to symptoms.

Dose: Tincture alone, 20 to 30 drops indicated by age and condition, every 2 to 3 hours.

Marrabium is an ingredient in practically all old-fashioned cough syrups and so innocent that it is an ingredient in a favorite candy.

In making an infusion, a teaspoonful of the powdered herb is added to a cup of boiling water; steep for half an hour; give a tablespoonful sweetened with a little honey, frequently.

Dosage: Tincture *Marrubium* alone, 5 to 40 drops in hot water as indicated.

INDIGO, WILD

Baptisia tinctoria

Common names: Rattlebush, Horse-fly Bush, Wild Indigo, Yellow Indigo.

Baptisia was once a household remedy in typhoid fever; later much prescribed by Eclectic and Physio-Medical physicians and continues to be much depended on by *Natura* physicians. Many physicians generally lost faith in it for the treatment of typhoid fever, until the Flower Hospital in New York made extensive experiments with it and found that faith in it was well-based.

Baptisia exerts a vital influence aiding in metabolism, in stimulating the elimination of accumulated waste in the body, and in encouraging normal organic activity. IT IS OF GREAT IMPORTANCE IN ALL SEPTIC AND DEGENERATIVE CONDITIONS, MANIFESTING THEMSELVES IN VARIOUS FORMS OF ULCERATION AND IMPORTANT IN SERIOUS ERUPTIVE DISEASES.

It is a dependable agent in ulcerative and mucous colitis and amoebic dysentery; both difficult conditions to cope with. In follicular tonsilitis and quinsy, it is indicated both as internal medication and as a gargle.

In false membraneous croup it helps to loosen the false membrane. It is a basic agent in the treatment of cracked nipples so frequently occurring at the beginning of nursing, best combined with non-alcoholic witch hazel and *Calendula*. In ulceration of the rectum, fluid extract of *Baptisia* should be combined with *Krameria*.

In all morbid, internal conditions a dependable formula is:

Tincture of Wild Indigo (*Baptisia tinctoria*)	2 to 20 drops
Tincture of Rhatany (*Krameria triandra*)	10 to 20 drops
Tincture of Coneflower (*Echinacea angustifolia*)	20 to 40 drops

In water every 2 to 4 hours depending on symptoms.

Dosage: Tincture *Baptisia* alone, 2 to 20 drops. *Dosage should be guarded.*

An infusion may be made with a teaspoonful of the powdered root, steeped in a pint of boiling water, 1 to 2 teaspoonsful every few hours, or according to condition. Half of this amount in a quart of slightly warm water in an enema in all septic or ulcerations of the rectum serves exceedingly well.

Specifically: *Baptisia* is indicated in the treatment of typhoid. Generally it is of great importance in the treatment of septic conditions of the blood, serious forms of prostration, muscular soreness, rheumatic and arthritic pains, in conditions where there is constriction of the chest, and general soreness of the body. It is well to combine with other remedies when there are chills associated with a temperature.

RED ROOT or JERSEY TEA

Ceanothus Americanus

Common names: New Jersey Tea, Wild Snowball, Red Root.

Ceanothus is considered as the spleen remedy, though it is probably second to *Chionanthus* in general practice.

Ceanothus is one of the few remedies which has a decided direct action on the spleen and is indicated also in all ailments where there is despondency and melancholy.

It is also astringent, an expectorant, sedative, anti-spasmodic, and anti-syphilitic, and may be combined with any other agents where these properties are required. It has proven useful in agents where these properties are required, in dyspepsia, especially of the nervous (mentally induced type) asthma, chronic bronchitis, whooping-cough, and consumption.

Special indication: Whenever there is a tendency during any ailment to despondency and melancholy and a tenderness to the touch over the region of the spleen, *Ceonothus* should from part of the formula or given alone in tincture form, though in domestic use an infusion was given.

Symptoms where the liver is involved with some type of dyspepsia, it is well combined with:

Tincture of Goldenseal (*Hydrastis canadensis*)	7 to 10 drops
Tincture of Fringe Tree (*Chiolanthus virginica*)	3 to 7 drops
Tincture of Jersey Tea (*Ceanothus americanus*)	10 to 20 drops

In water after meals and bedtime.

An infusion is made by steeping a teaspoon of the herb in cut or powdered form in a cup of boiling water, a teaspoon of this in water 3 or 4 times a day.

Dosage: Tincture *Ceanothus* alone, 10 to 20 drops in water 3 or 4 times a day.

KELP

Fucus vesiculosis

Kelp is neither a food nor a medicine except in the sense that it supplies mineral elements so essential to the normal functioning of the system in a form easily assimilated. It is a remedial agent in that it is rich in *Iodine* which the thyroid must have to properly function; therefore, it has a strong influence—is a sustainer—to both the nervous system and the brain, helping the brain to function normally. It is an essential during pregnancy.

The *Iodine* that is obtained from what are known as "kelp tablets" may be readily obtained from sea weed, one kind of which is used by many families for making blanc mange, a gelatin made with milk, honey, and flavoring highly prized by children.

Kelp is also rich in the mineral element *sodium,* so essential in the treatment of rheumatism and arthritis to keep the calcium in the system "liquefied"[1] and potassium, considered essential in the treatment of blood pollution and cancer.

Fucus is most helpful in the nourishment of the body, due to its ability to stimulate metabolism. It is a diuretic, in the sense that it helps to eliminate water imbalance (excess of water) from the system.

---

1. Not as yet generally conceded by the orthodox medical profession.

Valuable as it is, it cannot supplant thyroid (made from the fresh gland) for women in pregnancy, especially where there is a history of mental imbalance in the family history.

KNOTGRASS

Polyganum aviculare

Common names: Beggarweed, Pigweed, Red Robin.

Also known as the gravel remedy. Although Knotgrass is of much value in many ailments and considered as a domestic agent because it was long used for the purpose intended, its chief influence is on the bladder, and it has generally been used for the removal of stones from the bladder even after all other treatments had failed. It is not given to prevent the formation of stones, but to dissolve stones already formed. For this purpose it is best combined with Shave Grass three or more time a day, either in the infusion or tincture.

Tincture *Polygonum,* 10 to 20 drops combines well with the *Equisetum Arvenes* formula for the same purpose.

AMERICAN VALERIAN or LADY'S SLIPPER

Cypripedium pubescens

Common names: American Valerian, Umbel, Yellow Moccasin Flower, Noah's Ark.

"*Cypripedium* is adapted to atonic conditions and improves both the circulation and the nutrition of the nerve centers. As a remedy for nervous excitability or irritability not dependent upon organic lesions, it allays the irritation and with it, pain (if present) and produces a calm and tranquil condition of both body and mind. It is of special value in reflex functional disorders, or chorea, hysteria, nervous headache, insomnia low fevers, nervous unrest, hypochondria, and nervous depression accompanying stomach disorders. It is indicated in sleeplessness, neuralgia, and delirium, all due to atony; in menstrual irregularities, with despondency; mental depression from sexual over-indulgence; and in tendency to dementia at the climacteric."—*Dr. Thomas—Lloyd.*

In insomnia:

Tincture of Lady's Slipper (*Cypripedium pubescens*)	10 to 20 drops
Tincture of Passion Flower (*Pasiflora incarnata*)	10 to 20 drops

On retiring, repeat as necessary.

In despondency and a feeling of depression due to stomach disorders:

Tincture of Lady's Slipper (*Cypripedium pubescens*)	10 to 20 drops
Tincture of Common Chamomile (*Anthemis nobilis*)	8 to 20 drops

In water before meals, and on retiring.

Cypripedium is a mild acting tonic, diaphoretic and antispasmodic and a gentle nerve stimulant. It is especially important in the treatment of delicate children and women.

As a home remedy the root is best roughly ground, 5 tablespoons in a pint of boiling water; steep for an hour. One tablespoonful every hour, as needed. Dosage of tincture of *Cypripedium* alone, 5 to 30 drops according to age and severity of condition.

Specifically: Restlessness, chorea, hysteria, nervous depression, functional nervous disorders, inclination to neurosis, and dementia during climacterics.

LIFE ROOT

Senecio vulgaris

Common name: Groundsel, Common.

Life Root is also known as Squaw Weed, Golden Senecio, Female Regulator.

A woman's remedy: It was used as a household remedy and its common name of Life Root is an indication of the many different uses made of it.

It is an important agent in the various functional irregularities of women, especially during the menopause.

Senecio stimulates the pelvic organism, relieving engorgement. It strengthens flabby uterine ligaments. It removes pressure stemming from the perineum, bladder, and rectum, frequently following childbirth and during the menopause.

Senecio is both harmless and efficient in gynecological disorders such as dysmenorrhea, menorrhagia, atonic leukorrhea and other disturbances of the pelvic organism.

For diseases of men, it is an important agent in prostatic enlargement of the soft, boggy, atonic types.

Dosage: Tincture *Senecio* alone, 10 to 25 drops in water, three cf four times a day.

LILY-OF-THE-VALLEY

Convallaria magalis

Common name: May Lily.

A heart medicine. Substitute for digitalis, but is not toxic. It does upset the stomach.

The action of Convalarium is somewhat the opposite of *Cactus* and *Craetagus*. It increases the coronary circulation, promotes more vigorous and regular heart action correcting dyspnea and increasing urinary activity.

It combines well with *Echinacea* (Coneflower) and *Pytholacca* (Poke Root).

Dosage: Tincture *Convallarium* alone, 5 to 15 drops in water as required.

Specifically: *Convallaria* is indicated in distention of the heart ventricles, palpitation, dyspnea, and irregular heart beat. It is a heart tonic. It is of much value as a diuretic and combines well with other agents for that purpose, especially when there is an indication that the heart weakness is partially the cause. Dosage of the tincture, 5 to 20 drops in water and should always be well within limits, but may be given more frequently than three times a day if symptoms indicate it.

MARIGOLD

Calendula officinalis

Common names: Pot Marigold, Marybud, Holigold.

Calendula is the *Natura* physician's most reliable non-poisonous, non-toxic, non-irritating dressing for sores, burns, and wounds. It is an invaluable domestic aid and should be in the closet of every family where physicians are not always available.

"Old suppurating ulcers, sloughing sores, abscesses, non-malignant ulceration, excoriations, and chafing, burns and scalds are some of the conditions that may be permanently relieved. As a dressing to relieve uterine-catarrh, and as a wash to arrest offensive nasal discharge, it is an efficient agent."—*Dr. Niederkorn—Lloyd.*

"Useful in catarrhal and inflamed conditions of the mucous surfaces. A topical remedy in leukorrhea, simple ulcerations, pruritus ani, and vulvae, wounds, burns, traumatic injuries, and after surgical operations to promote healing."—*Dr. Anderson.*

Generally arnica is used where *Calendula* would be of much greater service.

For practically all wet dressings, including those to be applied by tampons to the cervix, the ideal combination is:

Tincture of Marigold (*Calendula officinalis*)	5 to 40 drops
Tincture of Goldenseal (*Hydrastis canadensis*)	7 to 12 drops
Tincture of Cranesbill (*Geranium maculatum*)	20 to 40 drops

The non-alcoholic tinctures should be used.

In malignant sores, whatever their nature, half an ounce of tincture *Echinacea* should be added.

Specifically: *Calendula* as a single remedy is of utmost importance in all irritated conditions of the mucous surfaces such as non-malignant ulcerations, leukorrhoea, all types of pruritus, for bruises and burns, and in almost every form of dressing for irritations.

MAY FLOWER

Pulsatilla

In chlorsis, due to its organic iron content, it is of great benefit, especially when there is nervousness. In neuralgia of the wandering, erratic type, it is indicated. In catarrhal affections such as mucous diarrhea and leukorrhoea it should be one of the agents employed In nervous and gastric sick-headache, it is equally beneficial.

Its greatest value, however, is in disorders of menstruation and spermatorrhoea. It has a decided influence upon the reproductive organism of both male and female. *It lessens sexual excitement, but at the same time increases sexual strength.*

Pulsatilla is a remedy of wide applicability, but more particularly *for those conditions in which the mind is a prominent factor. A gloomy mentality, a state of nerve depression and unrest, a disposition to brood over real or imagined trouble, a tendency to look on the dark side of life, sadness, mild restlessness, and a state of mental unrest generally denominated in broad terms nervousness* are factors in the condition of the patient requiring *Pulsatilla*. A *Pulsatilla* patient weeps easily, and the mind is inclined to wander—to be unsettled.

The pulse requiring *Pulsatilla* is weak, soft, and open, and the tissues have a tendency to dryness (except when the mucous tissues are discharging a thick, bland material), and about the orbits the parts appear contracted, sunken, and dark in color. The whole countenance and movements of the body depict sadness, moroseness, despondency, and lack of tone. *Hysteria of the mild and weeping form may be a symptom.* The whole condition is one of nervous depression, the nutrition of the nerve centers are at fault. With such symptoms, *Pulsatilla* may be confidently prescribed in the conditions and disorders enumerated. *Pulsatilla* may be given to produce sleep, when there is great exhaustion and opiates are inadmissible. If the insomnia depends upon determination of blood to the brain, *Pulsatilla* will not relieve, but when due to nervous exhaustion it is a prompter remedy to give rest, after which sleep obtains. Where sleep is disturbed by unpleasant dreams, and the patient awakens sad and languid, *Pulsatilla* should be given. *Pulsatilla* has a large field in troubles incident in the reproductive organs of both sexes. As an emmenagogue, it serves a useful purpose in amenorrhea in nervous and anemic subjects, with chilliness a prominent symptom. When menstruation is suppressed, tardy, or scanty from taking cold, or from emotional causes, *Pulsatilla* is the remedy. In dysmenorrhea, not due to mechanical causes, and with the above named nervous symptoms no remedy is more effective. Leukorrhoea, with free, thick, milky, or yellow, bland discharge and pain in the loins, and particularly in scrofulous individuals, calls for *Pulsatilla*. It is a remedy for mild forms of hysteria where the patient is weak and weeps easily, has fears of impending danger, and passes large quantities of clear, limpid urine, and menstruation is suppressed.

"The long-continued use of *Pulsatilla* as an intercurrent remedy is accredited with curative effects in uterine colic, but it is of no value during an attack. *Pulsatilla* frequently proves a good remedy in ovaritis and ovaralgia with tensive, tearing pain. Sluggish, ineffectual, and weak labor-pains are sometimes remedied by this drug. It is frequently a remedy for pain, when dependent on or associated with debility, and sometimes when due to acute inflammation. It is a leading remedy in *epididymitis* and orchitis, whether due to gonorrhoeal infection or to metastasis from mumps. The dark-red congested, enlarged, and sensitive testicle indicates it. It relieves the pains of *orchialgia,* and subdues *mammary* swelling from the metastasis of mumps. *Pulsatilla* increases sexual power, but lessens morbid sexual excitement. It is especially valuable in relieving urethral irritation and consequent spermatorrhoea and prostatorrhoea. In these troubles it overcomes the nervous apprehension so frequently a troublesome feature. It also alleviates the nervous irritability accompanying or produced by variocele. In gonorrhea, particularly of the chronic type, *Pulsatilla* is of value also in cases where the urethra membrane is swollen." Vol. 2, *American Dispensatory.*

Pulsatilla, though of special importance to the treatment of various past and especially of present day ailments with mental evolvements, is truly a woman's remedy, though it is of importance in the treatment of sex ailments in men.

Pulsatilla, though considered especially a sex-mental ailment remedy, has other important uses. It is indicated in catarrhal conditions of the ears frequently in children. Earache during colds and other minor and passing aural conditions respond to *Pulsatilla.*

Nasal catarrh so frequent in children, of an acute nature due to febrile affections, and the watery catarrhal discharges that may be persistent yield to its influence.

Pulsatilla should be taken *only under the direct care of a physician.*

Dosage: *Pulsatilla* alone, 1 to 3 drops in water every 2 or 3 hours or as indicated by severity of condition.

Specifically: *Pulsatilla* has been considered a sex remedy. It should be included in practically every formula for women's ailments *where there is a neurotic tendency. Pulsatilla* has a direct influence on the mental attitude (the brain) and the spinal cord, and upon the entire nervous system.

MOTHERWORT

Leonurus cardiaca

Leonurus is another of the *Natura* Physician's dependable remedies.

Leonurus is a composite agent and its real value is not generally understood. It is, in essence, a valuable bitter tonic and an actual stomachic of benefit in almost all stomach difficulties. It is a splendid nervine and of much value in dysmenorrhea, hysteria, palpitation of the heart, and urinary cramps, and may be used singly in all such cases, or in combination with other agents. It will inhibit, by removing the cause of, albumen in the urine, and the scanty muddy urine of typhoid, it is almost a specific, and it is valuable in many types of rheumatism.

Leonurus is a true tonic nervine. It is an agent especially strengthening to the heart—the indicated remedy in palpitation of the heart—useful in hysteria and in restlessness, pains peculiar to women, delirium tremens, and in some combinations of value in the treatment of affections of the liver.

It has frequently proven a matchless agent in rheumatism and sciatica, as well as in neuritis, due to its potency in the elimination of congestive material from the system.

Motherwort has been employed for time unknown as a domestic remedy, in the form of infusion. In long standing chronic conditions, a teaspoonful of the herb boiled in a pint of water until reduced by half, this divided into three portions to be taken one portion in the morning, one at noon, and one at night. Where there is pain or congestion, it should be taken in hot water.

In general practice it is best given in tablet form, three to four 3-grain tablets in hot or cold water according to condition.

Dosage: Tincture *Leonurus* alone, 9 to 15 drops in water 3 or more times a day.

Specifically: *Leonurus* in the smaller dosage should be prescribed for every woman during pregnancy. Experience has proven to physicians that it prevents frequent kidney complications during that period, especially albumen in the urine.

It combines well with all formulas for the various ailments so generally suffered by women during various periods in life. Its application should be carefully studied by the liberal and *Natura* physician to be fully informed of its use, as have been the women throughout the centuries, possibly even before its use by Indian women was made known to them.

MYRRH

Commiphora myrrha

Common name: Balsamodendon myrrha.

In morbid conditions, Myrrh is a remedy second only to *Echinacea*. It is usually spoken of as gum myrrh, although it contains very little gum, chiefly resin. In whatever form it is used, Myrrh will be found to be a powerful antiseptic having for thousands of years been used for preservative purposes, as well as a medicinal agent. It is generally administered as a tincture in water or syrup, although the powder may be given to equally good advantage. Two grains of the powdered Myrrh may be considered an average dose, best given combined with other indicated agents.

A small teaspoonful each of powdered Myrrh and Goldenseal to a pint of boiling water and a little ginger added will be found useful to weak stomach where the food is prone to ferment. Dose: A teaspoon every 2 hours.

Outwardly applied, Myrrh is invaluable for foul ulcers, bedsores, and all forms of gangrene and is mixed with powdered charcoal. Powdered Myrrh with *Hydrastis* may be sprinkled into indolent sores. Powdered Myrrh and Goldenseal, with a little borax, may be blown into the throat of persons suffering from diphtheria or other sore throat ailments. It will destroy the putrescence of the membranes and prevent blood absorption of toxins. Powdered Myrrh is a superior tooth powder, especially where the gums are tender and bleeding.

The compound tincture of Myrrh, known as Thomson Formula 6, is a powerful stimulant and antiseptic. It is unequalled as an antiseptic for foul ulcers and is superior, when diluted, to practically every other antiseptic in operative surgery. Internally, a few drops in a glass of water will prove a powerful stimulant in shock, collapse, prostration, and profound congestion.

Formula 6 may be quickly and readily made thus:

Tincture of Myrrh (*Commiphora myrrha*)	2 to 5 drops
(*Capsicum minimum*)	2 to 3 drops

In hot water as frequently as indicated by symptoms.

To add potency, tincture of Coneflower 10 drops, may be added.

Myrrh has been successfully employed in chronic diarrhoea and in diseases of the lungs and chest attended by a free expectoration and general debility. It is also well adapted to female complaints, when unattended by fever.

Applied to fresh wounds, the tincture of Myrrh excites healing action and lessens the liability to the occurrence of unhealthy inflammation. It is equally useful in old sores, ulcerated sore throat, running from the ears, aphthous sore mouth, spongy gums, and sore nipples.

The tincture of Myrrh is successfully employed to promote the exfoliation of bones. In sinus ulcers, and cavities that continue to discharge matter in consequence of a debilitated state of the vessels of the part, tincture of Myrrh injected into the cavity repeated daily, or even more often, will seldom fail to establish the inflammatory action necessary for the production of granulations and a union of the cavity. Where the parts are too sensitive to admit the tincture to be used undiluted, it may be combined with water, or better yet, Bayberry tea. In cases of scrofulous ulcers, white swellings, hip disease, and wherever there is a free discharge of matter from any reachable part of the body, and the system is in a relaxed condition, the use of Myrrh will prove beneficial.

After a vapor bath when the patient is rubbed dry, applying partly diluted tincture of Myrrh[2] affords a means of protection against cold, by strengthening and improving the condition of the skin. This practice is useful especially in cases where the skin is relaxed and the patient feeble, as in chronic bronchitis, consumption, chronic pleurisy, asthma, chronic rheumatism, chronic diarrhoea, marasmus, and in every other form of disease attended by general debility.

2. As it is now extremely difficult to procure pure grain alcohol for rubs after pack, steam or shower baths, the tincture of Myrrh should be used instead, thus assuring purity and harmlessness.

In deeply seated colds attended by a free expectoration of a thick yellowish secretion, the use of Thomson Formula 6 will be found highly beneficial.

An external application of Thomson Formula 6, i.e., compound tincture of Myrrh and *Capsicum,* has been found useful in rheumatism, neuralgia, and like ailments. To help bring about relaxation, an equal amount of tincture *Lobelia* may be added. In applying the compound for the relief of dropsy, night-sweats, consumption, and in all diseases where the skin is relaxed, *Lobelia* need not be added.

The compound tincture may be applied to great advantage in sprains, bruises, fresh cuts, indolent ulcers, gangrene, and as a preventive to mortification both internally and externally.

In that much and rightly dreaded condition foreshadowing mastoiditis where there is running of the ear or where this can be induced, there is no safer or more successful method for the possible relief of the condition, than the frequent syringing of the ear with:

Tincture of Myrrh (*Commiphora myrrha*)	5 drops
Tincture of Coneflower (*Echinacea angustifolia*)	5 drops

Mix with half ounce of warm water: 5 drops in the ear 2 or 3 times a day, lightly massaging the area around the ear after drops are used and warmth applied over the ear.

Dosage of tincture of Myrrh alone, 2 to 5 drops.

Specifically: Myrrh stimulates indolent ulcers and eczema when applied externally. The undiluted tincture is applied to ulcerated gums, aphthous patches, and relaxed conditions of the vulva, pharynx, and in ptyalism.

Internally, it is employed in bronchitis and sometimes in tuberculosis. Atonic dyspepsia is often favorably influenced by Myrrh combined with bitters. In amenorrhea, it is combined with other indicated agents.

PASSION FLOWER

Passiflora incarnata

Passiflora should be given in all feverish conditions where there is extreme nervousness and lack of sleep. It is quieting and soothing to the nervous system. The *Natura* physician refuses to give drugs that are habit forming. *Passiflora* takes the place of narcotics.

"*Passiflora* is helpful for nervousness, when not due to pain. Where there is a state of unrest, agitation, worry, and exhaustion; the patient does not sleep; there is cerebral excitement and a marked tendency toward convulsion, particularly in the young, as evidenced by muscular twitching. When convulsions are accompanied or preceded by the foregoing, *Passiflora* is a valuable agent. It is useful in controlling asthenic insomnia, particularly of childhood and old people. When in typhoid and other dynamic fevers, the patient is extremely restless and excitable and cannot sleep, this agent will give rest and slowly produce a remarkably natural and refreshing sleep. It is especially valuable for asthenic conditions; when these are present it tones the sympathetic nervous system, improving the circulation and nutrition of the nerve centers."—*Dr. Neiderkorn—Lloyd.*

Passiflora is an antispasmodic indicated in insomnia generally, many types of neuroses, some forms of asthma, and acute (temporary) mania. In these cases 30 to 60 drops of the tincture are given frequently. It is a safe remedy to give to restless children small doses of 3 to 10 drops in water every 30 minutes until there is relief.

Passiflora is considered by the *Natura* physician as a mild antispasmodic and soporific in infantile spasms and restlessness in low fevers, and in reflex nervous excitement and should be prescribed instead of bromides.

Passiflora is best prescribed in the form of tincture or tablets.

Dosage: Tincture of *Passiflora* alone, 15 to 60 drops in water according to age and condition as frequently as necessary.

Specifically: *Passiflora* is the "opium" (non-poisonous and not dangerous) of the true *Natura* physician. It is an antispasmodic and mild soporific. It is indicated in asthenic insomnia, in some cases of infantile spasms, and also in the restlessness and insomnia of low fevers. It is given by physico-medicalists in cases usually placed under bromide medication.

PEPPERMINT

Mentha piperita

Peppermint, though not of the same type of herb, is much of the same nature as Horehound and Spearmint and is well combined with them in making an infusion or syrup. Peppermint has an additional virtue, it is of much value in the colic and cramps of children. Infusion, made in the same manner, by itself or in combination with Horehound and Spearmint, and given in the same dosage for colic and cramps, always in hot water as frequently as necessary.

Dosage: Tincture *Mentha Piperita* alone, 10 to 50 drops according to age and severity of attack.

PIPSISSEWA
PRINCE'S PINE—CHIMAPHILIA UMBELIATA

Chimaphila umbellata

Common names: Ground Holly, Prince's Pine, and its most familiar name "Winter Green." Not to be confused with Wintergreen (*Gaultheria procumbens*).

The Dropsy remedy. Infusions of Wintergreen were a domestic remedy long before tinctures, and the oil was part of medical practice. Pipsissewa is a diuretic, tonic, alternative, and an astringent. It is of great value in scrofula and chronic rheumatism. In diseases of the kidneys, especially dropsy, it is the *Natura* physician's standby.

In scrofula and other blood diseases it is best combined with other agents such as yellow dock, dandelion root, and others of like nature.

In dropsy:

Tincture of Pipsissewa (*Chimaphila umbellata*)	2 to 15 drops
Tincture of Poplar Bark (*Populus tremuloides*)	10 to 15 drops

Three or four times a day, according to condition—always in plenty of water. The same combination may be given successfully in conditions when the urine is scanty, and containing offensive and non-offensive pus, or pus and blood mixed. When the urine is scalding or burning, in chronic urethral and prostatic irritations, chronic relaxation of the bladder, and chronic prostatitis with catarrh of the bladder, it is of great value in skin diseases, of benefit in gonorrheal rheumatism.

In folk or domestic usage the combination of agents was made into an infusion, but it is best given in the tincture:

Tincture of Pipsissewa (*Chimaphila umbellata*)	2 to 15 drops
Tincture of Poke Root (*Phytolacca decandra*)	2 to 10 drops
Tincture of Prickly Ash (*Xanthoxylum americanum*)	5 to 20 drops
Tincture of Stickwort (*Agrimonia Eupatoria*)	10 to 30 drops

In water, three or four times a day.

Dosage: Tincture of Pipsissewa, 2 to 15 drops in water as frequently as required.

PLEURISY ROOT

Asclepias tuberose

Common names: Butterfly-Weed, Wind Root, Tuber Root, Canada Root.

A diaphoretic that is always safe and certain in its action and when given in sufficiently large doses in hot water it is the ideal medication in pneumonia and pleurisy. In these acute conditions it must be combined with another agent such as *Scutellaria*. *Asclepias* should always be administered in the form of a hot infusion or the tincture given in water hot as the patient can drink. It is an entirely safe sweating agent and should be used freely until free perspiration is secured. In high temperature, especially in pneumonia, where quick action is desired the regular dose should be administered every half hour or even more frequently. Once free perspiration has been established, the dosage may be decreased by giving less frequently, but always in warm water, until the temperature is near normal and the lungs free from congestion.

"*Asclepias* is the diaphoretic and is associated with a sedative when an increased action of the skin is required.

"*Asclepias* has a decided influence over serous and mucous membranes, hence it becomes exceedingly useful as an associate remedy in pleurisy. Alone it is a decided remedy for catarrhal affections of the pulmonary and gastro-intestinal tracts when due to colds. For these purposes it is especially adapted to the stomach and bowel disorders of children exhibited by weakness, mucous discharges, and gastric irritability, with general nervous unrest. It is a remedy for vaso-disturbances in the parts supplied by the bronchial arteries and is a prompt remedy for intercostal pain.

"It is especially a child's remedy, being feeble in its action in small doses, though quite certain. When freely given, it is one of the most certain diaphoretics we have. Even in small doses of one drop, it will markedly increase the true secretions from the skin."—*Dr. Feller—Lloyd.*

In the onset of colds, give 5 to 15 drops of the tincture of *Asclepias* in hot water, and 3 grains of Capsicum, every hour until the whole person is warm as indicated. While taking this remedy in hot water or as an infusion, chills must be carefully avoided.

Children may be given 1 to 5 drops in hot water depending on age and condition. If very restless, add same amount of *Scutellaria*.

In pneumonia and acute pleurisy give:

Tincture of Pleurisy Root (*Asclepias tuberose*)	15 to 40 drops
Tincture of Skullcap (*Scutellaria Lateriflora*)	2 to 20 drops

Every hour, or more frequently, until a free perspiration is established; then less frequently, and as soon as the lungs are free an active stimulant like *Capsicum* should be taken, followed by a tonic of the nature of *Hydrastis*. Children, 3 to 10 drops, depending on age and condition.

In peritonitis give:

Tincture of Pleurisy Root (*Asclepias tuberose*)	20 to 30 drops
Tincture of Coneflower (*Echinacea angustifolia*)	2 to 30 drops
Tincture of Indian Tobacco (*Lobelia inflata*)	3 to 10 drops

Every 1 or 2 hours in cool water. If the temperature becomes subnormal, Cayenne Pepper in 2 to 4 grain doses every hour.

In all acute congested conditions of the lungs, *Asclepias* is the indicated remedy. Boneset may be substituted for *Scutellaria* when this agent is not procurable.

Dosage: Tincture *Asclepias,* 5 to 40 drops every 3 hours or more frequently depending on age and condition.

Infusion: 1 teaspoon cut or powdered herb in a teacup of boiling water, steep for half an hour. Every 3 or 4 hours, for adults; in proportion for children.

Specifically: Dryness of the respiratory mucous membranes, especially when associated with a dry and slight fever—a condition met with in many respiratory ailments.

POKE ROOT

Phytolacca decandra

Poke Root has a long history of usefulness in medicine. It has been a household remedy for time beyond memory, and though toxic in too large an amount there is no record of its ever having caused harmful results, indicating that the housewives using it understood both its value and its limitations.

Phytolacca is an alternative, a purgative, and an emetic. The housewife generally depended on *Lobelia* (Indian Tobacco) as an emetic and on Poke Root as a purgative.

In large doses it is a heart depressant and reduces blood pressure, and it is useful for that purpose but should not be long continued.

It is an alterative; it stimulates metabolism, hence useful in medication for undernourishment. It helps greatly in detoxicating the system from poisonous congestions.

It is valuable in the treatment of rheumatism, lymphatic engorgement, and toxins in the blood.

It is a dependable agent in the treatment of mammillary swelling from which so many women suffer following childbirth, making nursing impossible. In such cases, a mixture of *Phytolacca,* 3 parts to 1 part of glycerine, will abort the swelling at its beginning, or where suppuration has taken place it will help in drainage and bring about granulation.

Specifically: *Phytolacca* is indicated and should be combined in the formulas for throat conditions, especially when the membrane is dark in color, tonsils swollen, shooting pains through the ear. With difficulty in swallowing it should be thought of at the first indication of irritation or inflammation of the throat and combined with other agents in the treatment. It should also form a part of the formulas in the treatment of chronic rheumatism and arthritis.

Its usefulness in costiveness has been proven throughout time.

Dosage: Tincture of *Phytolacca* alone, 2 to 5 drops as frequently as indicated by symptoms.

POND LILY, WHITE

Nymphaea Odorata

Common names: Sweet-Scented Water Lily, Sweet Water Lily.

The non-alcoholic tincture is an excellent remedy for cold sores of the mouth, scrofulous sores, as well as for purulent ophthalmia.

Nymphaea Odorata is an excellent agent in practically all cankerous conditions and in complaints of the bowels.

Locally, for leukorrhea and in direct tampon applications or packing for prolapsus uteri, ulceration of the cervix, and relaxed vagina, it has few superiors.

It gives best results when combined with:

Non-alcoholic Tincture of Goldenseal (*Hydrastis canadensis*)   1 ounce
Non-alcoholic Tincture of Marigold (*Calendula officinale*)   1 ounce
Non-alcoholic Tincture of White Pond Lily (*Nymphaea odorata*)   1 ounce

Only the non-alcoholic tinctures should be used. The same combination diluted may be used as a wash for sore eyes. With the addition of one-quarter ounce tincture of Myrrh to the formula, this combination is excellent for sore breasts, a painful and annoying condition which many women suffer and which does not respond to the average treatment. *Nymphaea* has the virtue of being non-poisonous and non-irritating and may readily be applied frequently by nursing mothers.

POPLAR

Populus tremuloides

Common names: White Poplar, American Aspen, Quaking Aspen.

Poplar bark, as well as the leaves, have long been used domestically as an infusion by Thomsonian, physio-medical and *Natura* physicians as a bitters to restore the digestive disturbances.

Used either as an infusion or the tincture, it will relax the system, relieve headache due to the liver or stomach conditions, relieve many other complaints caused by faulty digestion.

It is of much value in obstruction of the urine when not due to prostatitis and weakness in the loins, and for those of a consumptive constitution it should be given freely.

In chronic diarrhoea, chronic dysentery, and cholera infantum it is a tonic rather than a stimulant.

Populus is clearly indicated in uterine, vaginal, and anal weaknesses.

It is most effective when combined with *Uva-Ursi:*

Tincture of Quaking Aspen (*Populus tremuloides*)	2 to 15 drops
Tincture of Upland Cranberry (*Arctostaphylos Uvi-Ursi*)	10 to 20 drops

In water three to four times a day.

Tincture of *Populus* alone, 2 to 15 drops in water as indicated.

Infusion: 1 teaspoon of either, or both, in a cup of boiling water, steep half an hour, cool; take two or more times a day.

RASPBERRY

Rubus Strigosus

Common name: Wild Red Raspberry.

Known as the children's remedy, long used in domestic practice as a remedy in the bowel complaint of children.

Strigosus is a mild, pleasant, soothing, diffusive, stimulating, astringent tonic, allaying nausea, sustaining the nerves, and toning the mucous membranes.

It is a splendid agent in the relief of urethral irritation and is soothing to the kidneys, urinary tract, and ducts. It is dependable to sustain the uterus and stop hemorrhages. In such cases it should be combined with equal parts *Myrica:*

Tincture of Raspberry (*Rubus Idaeus*)	5 to 20 drops
Tincture of Bayberry (*Myrica cerifera*)	10 to 40 drops

In water three to four times a day.

For the relief of urethral irritations, kidney infections, chronic dysentery, and hemorrhages:

Tincture of Witch Hazel (*Hamamelis virginiana*)	10 to 40 drops
Tincture of Goldenseal (*Hydrastis canadensis*)	7 to 12 drops
Tincture of Raspberry (*Rubus Idaeus*)	7 to 10 drops

In water according to symptoms as frequently as required.

Mothers generally have greater faith in the infusion than the tinctures: 1 teaspoon of the bark and roots added to a cup of boiling water, steep one-half hour or more; strain. One-half teaspoon every 2 hours or more frequently. Continue until effective.

As a douche in leukorrhoea and as an enema for severe dysentery, 30 drops of *Hydrastis,* 1 tablespoon of non-alcoholic Hamamelis added to a quart of cool water. Repeat as necessary.

Dosage: Tincture of Raspberry *Strigosus* alone, 30 to 60 drops in water as required.

RHATANY
Krameria

Krameria is not generally known even to the profession, nevertheless, it is one of the most important agents in the treatment of typhoid fever and in all conditions where there is chronic inflammation of the alimentary system such as enteritis, gastritis, proctitis, and other ailments of similar nature.

Krameria is useful in the treatment of diarrhoea, including amoebic dysentery and in ulcerated colitis as direct medication via the enema.

Krameria is indicated in all diseases in which *Baptisia* (Indigo) is prescribed:

Tincture of Rhatany (*Krameria triandra*)	10 to 30 drops
Tincture of Wild Indigo (*Baptisia tinctoria*)	2 to 20 drops

In water every 2 or 3 hours. Dosage and frequency to age and condition. *Dosage should be guarded.*

In conditions where pus is present, as in ulceration, mucous colitis, amoebic dysentery, and disease of like nature, several drops of *Myrrh* should be added.

RHEUMATISM ROOT
Dioscarea Villosa

Common name: Wild Yam.

The rheumatism remedy. This is another of the long used household or domestic remedies used in the treatment of rheumatism and later adopted by the Eclectic and Physio-Medical physicians. It is an alternative and stimulates the removal of accumulated wastes and congestions in the system, especially in the joints.

It is best when combined with:

Tincture of Burdock Root (*Arctium Lappa*)	10 to 40 drops
Tincture of Black Cohosh (*Cimicifuga racemosa*)	2 to 15 drops
Tincture of Motherwort (*Lonurus cardiaca*)	10 to 20 drops
Tincture of Rheumatism Root (*Dioscarea Villosa*)	20 to 40 drops

In water 3 or 4 times a day.

Dosage: Tincture *Dioscarea* alone, 10 to 30 drops in water 3 or 4 times a day according to symptoms.

SCULLCAP, VIRGINIAN

Scutellaria Lateriflora

Common names: Hoodwort, Side-flowering Scullcap, Mad Weed, Mad-Dog Scullcap.

Scullcap is best known to country people as Hoodwort or Mad-Dog Weed.

From time memorial it has been used for them in feverishness in children to induce perspiration and reduce temperature.

It has been, and continues to be, successfully used as a female remedy for cramps and severe pain caused by suppressed menstruation due to colds. In hysteria due to ovarian or uterine origin, when given in conjunction with Pennyroyal as a tea, it is decidedly beneficial.

Scullcap is one of the most reliable tonic nervines and best used in the form of an infusion from the herb or in practice the tincture in hot water.

Combined with *Capsicum* and *Hydrastis* there is no substitute in weaknesses of the heart:

Tincture of Scullcap (*Scutellaria Lateriflora*)	3 to 15 drops
Tincture of Goldenseal (*Hydrastis canadensis*)	7 to 10 drops
Tincture of Cayenne Pepper (*Capsicum frutescens*)	2 to 4 drops

In warm water as often as required.

In irritable, nervous conditions, *Scutellaria* should be combined with:

Tincture of Lady's Slipper (*Cypripedium pubescens*)   10 to 20 drops
Tincture of Scullcap (*Scutellaria Lateriflora*)   2 to 15 drops

In water, every 2 to 4 hours in cold water as required.

A popular name given Scullcap long ago—mad weed or mad-dog weed—is because of one of its former uses in preventing or curing hydrophobia and the bites of poisonous snakes in combination with:

Tincture of Coneflower (*Echinacea angustifolia*)   15 to 30 drops
Tincture of Scullcap (*Scutellaria Lateriflora*)   2 to 15 drops

In water in doses as frequently as indicated.

Scullcap is a dependable sedative. It is invaluable in undue sexual desire and may be given freely and persistently without the slightest harm. In such cases it is best taken in the form of a tea made from the herb itself. If this is nonprocurable, use the tincture in hot water.

"*Scutellaria,* by its action through the cerebro-spinal centers, is a most valuable remedy controlling nervous irritation, calming hysterical excitement, and relieving functional heart troubles where cardiac action is irregular. In restlessness and excitement with insomnia following prolonged application to business, long sickness, or physical exhaustion it is most useful. When given in hot drinks it acts more quickly and also brings on diaphoresis. In treating heavy drinkers who wish to give up the habit, I know of nothing better than *Scutellaria*. It steadies and sobers the patient and brings on sleep and appetite."—*Dr. Fearn—Lloyd*.

In insomnia or exhaustion, whether from excessive application to business or due to alcoholics, give:

Tincture of Scullcap (*Scutellaria Lateriflora*)   2 to 12 drops
Tincture of Passion Flower (*Passiflora incarnata*)   15 to 40 drops

In water every 3 hours or more frequently depending on age and condition.

Dosage: Tincture *Asclepias* alone, 3 to 12 drops in water as indicated.

Infusion: One teaspoonful cut or powdered herb steeped in a teacup of boiling water, steep half an hour. Every 3 or 4 hours for adults, in proportion for children.

Specifically: *Scutellaria* is a sedative and tonic nervine. It has a direct action on the cerebro-spinal centers, controls nervous irritation, relieves restlessness and insomnia in fevers.

SHAVE GRASS

Equisetum arvense
Equisetum hyemale
Equisetum maximum
Equisetum sylvaticum

Common name: Horsetails.

Commonly known as the gravel remedy.

Shave Grass has long been used and is indicated in most kidney and bladder ailments, especially in painful urination and when blood is present in the urine.

It is useful as a compress in the treatment of old sores where foul-smelling pus is present in combination with comfrey and myrrh.

Internally in all indicated conditions:

Tincture of Shave Grass (*Equisetum arvense*)	5 to 20 drops
Tincture of Couch Grass (*Triticum repens*)	20 to 40 drops
Tincture of Corn Silk (*Stigmata Maydis*)	10 to 20 drops

In water 3 or more times a day as required by condition.

Dosage: Tincture *Equisetum* alone, 5 to 20 drops in water, 3 times a day. As a domestic remedy, it is still much used in infusion: One teaspoon of Shave Grass in a cup of boiling water, steep one-half an hour, allow to cool. One tablespoonful 4 or more times a day as required.

SPEARMINT

Mentha viridis

Spearmint is a companion to Horehound, and like Horehound has always been, and continues to be, a family remedy. It combines well with Spearmint, and for feverishness in children should be given in infusion or the tincture in hot water.

In the extreme restlessness of feverish children, it should also be given in enemas.

Spearmint, in hot infusion, will help produce perspiration and the flow of urine in high fevers. In pleurisy and pneumonia it is a splendid agent when combined with *Asclepias* and *Scutellaria* or other agents. The formula for the combination is the same as with Horehound. Spearmint has been called the emesis remedy because it will stop vomiting when other remedies are ineffective.

Dosage: Tincture *Mentha Viridis* alone, 10 to 50 drops in hot water according to age and condition.

Infusion is made by steeping a teaspoon of the herb in a cup of hot water for one-half an hour; 1 tablespoonful frequently.

Like *Marrubium,* it combines well with practically all fever, cold, and cough agents.

SQUAW VINE
Mitchella repens

Common names: Partridgeberry, One-Berry, Checkerberry, Winter Clover, Deerberry, Hive Vine.

Most important function: For ages past, the American Indian women have used Squaw Vine as a tea or infusion all during pregnancy to assure proper development of the child and render parturition both safe and easy, and at the same time develop lactation.

The Physio-Medical and *Natura* physician have learned by experience that *Mitchella* has other important virtues, but use it principally for this purpose.

Mitchella, besides being a parturient, a diuretic, and an astringent, in practice it is generally best known as a uterine tonic, to relieve congestion of the uterus and ovaries. It will help restore the menstrual function and relieve menorrhagia, amenorrhea, and dysmenorrhea. The continued use of *Mitchella* will control unpleasant nervous reflexes during pregnancy and is one of the reasons that many women use it continually during the period of gestation. *Mitchella* stimulates lactation and aids in normal recovery after confinement. Its use should be continued during the entire period of nursing.

In domestic use an infusion or tea was made. One teaspoon of Squaw Vine in a cup of boiling water, steep one-half an hour, let cool before drinking. On an average, 2 or 3 cups a day throughout pregnancy and nursing.

Dosage: Tincture *Mitchella* alone, as a general medication, 5 to 15 drops three times a day. The most desirable way to give it during pregnancy and nursing is in tablet form, two to three, 3 grain tablets three times a day.

The berries crushed into a pulp and added to tincture of Myrrh are highly potent as a cure for sore nipples. Another method is to boil leaves and berries in a pint of water until the pint is reduced to 2 ounces, then add one-quarter ounce of tincture of Myrrh and an ounce of glycerine. Apply frequently. The berries used for an infusion are excellent in the treatment of dysentery when occurring during pregnancy. In general practice tincture should be used.

STARGRASS

Aletris Farinosa

Common name: Ague Root, Crow Corn, True Unicorn Root, Colic Root.

The woman's remedy. Compatible with, and well combines with, Squaw Vine and Pleurisy Root during entire period of gestation.

Stargrass is a gentle stimulating and toning agent influencing the female generative organism. In dysmenorrhoea it stimulates and tones the uterus to normal action and relieves pain. In menorrhagia it controlls excessive flow. It is one of the best preventives to miscarriage and is associated with vitamin E. It is highly desirable to prescribe it during the entire period of pregnancy together with Squaw Vine and Milkwort:

Tincture of Stargrass (*Aletris farinosa*)	10 to 40 drops
Tincture of Squaw Vine (*Mitchella repens*)	5 to 15 drops
Tincture of Milkwort (*Polygala vulgaris*)	1 to 15 drops

In water 3 or 4 times a day.

Dosage: Tincture of Stargrass alone, 15 to 40 drops in water as frequently as required.

In menorrhagia, dysmenorrhea and pain due to menstrual dysfunctioning:

Tincture of Stargrass (*Aletris farinosa*)	20 to 40 drops
Tincture of Black Haw (*Vibrurnum opulus*)	5 to 20 drops
Tincture of Blue Cohosh (*Caulophyllum thalictroides*)	5 to 15 drops
Tincture of Squaw Vine (*Mitchella repens*)	5 to 15 drops

In hot water as required.

Specifically: This combination of natural agents has proven exceptionally successfull in the treatment of ailments to which many women are subject. It is dependable and free from after effects.

SUNDEW

Drosea rotundifolia

The whooping cough remedy. Though long a household remedy for this annoying and often serious affliction, it found a welcome place in the practice of the Eclectic, Physio-Medical and later liberal and *Natura* physicians.

Drosea is especially valuable in controlling the spasms and cough present generally in whooping cough.

Sundew is also indicated in laryngitis and for tobacco cough. It is best combined with:

Tincture of Sundew (*Drosera Rotundifolia*)	2 to 5 drops
Tincture of Queen's Root (*Stillingia Silvatica*)	1 to 40 drops
Tincture of Passion Flower (*Passiflora incarnata*)	3 to 10 drops

In water as frequently as necessary.

Dosage: Tincture *Drosea* alone, 3 to 6 drops in water as indicated.

Specifically: Frequent violent spasms of coughing and dry throat associated with a deep, hoarse voice. Feeling of oppression in the chest, worse at night.

TOUCH-ME-NOT

Impatiens aurea
Impatiens biflora

Common names: Balsam Weed, Balsam Jewelweed, Pale Touch-Me-Not.

As its name "touch-me-not" implies, it is a warning against ivy (rhus) poisoning which may be easily contracted by a mere touch. As balsam it is soothing and healing in weeping eczema—blisters formed and opened.

In domestic use the fresh plant is crushed and applied. An infusion may be made by steeping several ounces of the plant or powder in 8 ounces of boiling water for half an hour, strain and it is ready for use. Dusting with the powder is also effective.

It can also be made into an ointment by slowly boiling the fresh plant in lard, any strength desired, or heating the lard and mixing the powder with it. Either infusion, powder or salve may be applied to the poisoned areas of eczema.

The salve is of much value in treating bruises, wounds, ulcerated conditions, and hemorrhoids.

TURTLE-HEAD

Chelone Glabra

Common name: Lesser Centuary, Bitter Herb, Balmony.

Chelone is a splendid agent in the treatment of common dyspepsia and may be used freely for atonic conditions. It influences the liver favorably and will combine well with *Hydrastis* and *Chionanthus*. It is a moderate stimulating cholagogue. It is of service in the treatment of chronic jaundice on account of its action on the bile. As a mild hepatic tonic, it does well in convalescence from fevers and other diseases where the liver is involved. In malassimilation, it is one of the best agents, and it does good service in freeing the system of stomach worms. In general debility it serves as a tonic.

Combined with diuretics, its tonic powers are exerted on the kidneys; and in dropsy where there is chronic, hepatic, and gastric torpor, the influence of this agent is excellent.

In jaundice, malnutrition and all conditions where the sufferer consumes a sufficient amount of food but is not fully nourished by it, the best combination is:

Tincture of Fringe Tree (*Chiolanthus virginica*)	5 to 10 drops
Tincture of Turtle-Head (*Chelone glabra*)	10 to 20 drops
Tincture of Goldenseal (*Hydrastis canadensis*)	7 to 10 drops

In a glass of water before each meal.

This formula is excellent, when there is a general deficiency of bile *indicated by light colored stool*. It is also indicated for children when this condition exists over an extended period. Dose: According to age.

For stomach and intestinal worms, the dose is from 3 to 40 drops, depending upon the age of the person.

Dosage: Tincture *Chelone* alone, 10 to 20 drops, in water 3 or 4 times a day.

UNICORN ROOT, FALSE

Chamaelirium luteum

Common name: Helonias.

A miscarriage preventive remedy. False Unicorn Root is considered a woman's remedy.

The *Natura* physician uses it frequently singly, or in combination with other agents, during women's menopause. It is of much value in practically all cases where there is pelvic atony, a sense of pressure in the ovarian tubes and sacrum, and irritation of the bladder. Especially valuable in nervousness, mental confusion, neurotic tendency, and general apathy.

Where there is a history of miscarriage, it is of value either singly or with other agents indicated and in association with vitamin E.

Helonias is a tonic valuable in functional irritability, poor assimilation, nervous dyspepsia—usually called nervous indigestion—anemia, and anorexia.

Dose of the tincture, 10 to 40 drops in water 3 or 4 times a day or more frequently according to symptoms.

Dosage: Tincture *Serpentaris* alone, 1 to 20 drops in water as indicated.

While the infusion has been extensively used as a household remedy in districts where the plant is plentiful and the services of a physician not always available, it should be prescribed only by a physician when available.

VIRGINIA SNAKEROOT

Aristolochia serpentaria

Common names: Red River Snakeroot, Texas Snakeroot, Sangrel, Sangree Root.

Virginia Snakeroot is stimulating to the mucous membrane throughout, but should be given only in small doses. In languid and sluggish conditions of the organism, it activates promptly and fully, and for this reason it is valuable in confinement cases when the feet are cold and there is a general receding of the blood from the surface.

In eruptive diseases, before the appearance of the full eruption, it is excellent in small doses in hot water. In these cases it will do well combined with Burdock:

Tincture of Virginia Snakeroot (*Aristolochia serpentaria*)   1 to 20 drops
Tincture of Burdock (*Arctium Lappa*)   10 to 30 drops

In warm water every few hours until free eruptions.

Serpentaria's influence is primarily to induce blood circulation toward the surface, but soon its influence is felt by the whole arterial system, and the heart's impulse becomes stronger and fuller. By its stimulating action upon the arterial circulation, the whole nervous system is aroused through its influence. Even the uterus feels the effect, and its use is valuable for the relief of menstruation suppressed by colds. In these cases, 5 to 10 drops of the tincture is more effective given in hot Pennyroyal tea.

Cold preparations, whether of the infusion or the tincture in cold water, will favorably influence action of the kidneys and relieve congestion and renal torpor.

WHITE COHOSH

Actaea alba

A woman's remedy. A nervine and dependable emmenagogue in the hand of a capable physician.

Indicated in the treatment of nervous, asthenic women. Its strongest affect is upon pelvice plexus in the treatment of amenorrhea, dysmenorrhea, and ovarian cramps or spasms, relieving pelvic congestion and irritation.

It is well combined with:

Tincture of Blue Cohosh (*Caulophyllum thalictroides*)   2 to 5 drops
Tincture of Black Cohosh (*Cimicifuga racemosa*)   1 to 10 drops
Tincture of Squaw Weed (*Senecio aureus*)   3 to 5 drops
Tincture of Black Haw (*Viburnum opulus*)   5 to 10 drops
Tincture of White Cohosh (*Actea alba*)   1 to 5 drops

In water every 2 to 4 hours depending on condition.

Dosage: Tincture of Actea alone, 2 to 5 drops as frequently as required.

Specifically: Actea is especially indicated in chorea, hysteria, emotional irritability, mental depression, neurotic tendencies, and especially so when due to menstrual irregularities.

WITCH HAZEL

Hamamelis virginiana

Common name: Winterbloom, Snapping Hazelnut, Spotted Alder.

Witch Hazel is another of the ageless household or domestic remedies said to have been used by the Indians for various irritations (for which it is still best known). The non-alcoholic preparation is now easily obtainable and is most satisfactorily used for this purpose.

The infusion is the most valuable in hemoptysis, hematemesis, and other forms of bleeding, as well as in diarrhea, dysentery, and excessive mucous discharge. It is of value also in incipient tuberculosis. However, when the fresh herb is not obtainable, then the tincture (non-alcoholic when obtainable) is satisfactory and may be given in cold or hot water according to the symptoms. There is hardly an inflamed condition, internally or externally, where it may not be prescribed with benefit. In sore mouth, inflamed eyes, burns and bruises it is equally soothing.

With Hops or Flaxseed the herb may be made into a poultice for external inflammations, swellings, and tumors of a painful character.

An ointment made with lard and Witch Hazel, White Oak Bark, and Apple Tree Bark, ground Horse Chestnuts, together with burnt cork is excellent in the treatment of hemorrhoids.

It may be applied full strength to painful tumors, external inflammation of prolapsus ani and uteri, leukorrhea, gleet, and ophthalmia. As an enema in the treatment of dysentery and diarrhea. When the rectum and large bowel are inflamed, nothing will bring the quick relief that witch hazel and cold water will.

Witch Hazel is of much value in the treatment of children's various "summer complaints." Dosage: 5 to 30 drops of the tincture in water as often as indicated.

A simple soothing toning agent is composed of:

Tincture of Witch Hazel (*Hamamelis virginiana*)	10 to 40 drops
Tincture of Goldenseal (*Hydrastis canadensis*)	5 to 40 drops
Tincture of Raspberry (*Rubus Idaeus*)	5 to 40 drops

In water. This allays nausea, sustains the nervous system, tones the mucous membranes, splendid in chronic or acute dysentery and diarrhea, reduces all urinary inflammation, and is frequently a cure for gleet.

Dosage: Tincture of Witch Hazel alone, 10 to 60 drops in cold water as often as necessary.

9.

THE MEDICINES OF OUR FOREFATHERS

The agents listed were the medicines of our forefathers, many of whom had no other source of treatment.

Among the best known and most effective were those first known by the Indians. In turn, the early physicians learned of them, and they became part of their medical practice.

A great many of these agents continue to be used regularly by liberal physicians who still adhere to the practice with the medicines of nature, *God-given and God-commanded* NATURE'S HEALING AGENTS; an increasing number who had changed to chemical agents are returning to their use, and they are being increasingly used as family remedies.

The preparation of infusions and dosages of tinctures is given and, in some instances, the combinations of herbs for infusions.

BARBERRY

Berberis Vulgaris

The liver and spleen remedy as well a blood disease and tuberculosis remedy.

Berberis is indicated in the chronic ills of the stomach and the early stages of tuberculosis. It also is frequently prescribed in the catarrhal conditions of the bronchial tubes.

It is well employed as a tonic in all debilitated conditions, convalescence from serious ailments, and in various skin diseases due to digestive disturbances. It combines well with almost all agents for the treatment or relief of liver and spleen ailments, especially with *Hydrastis* and *Chionanthus*.

Best given in the tincture, 5 to 10 drops before meals.

120

BARLEY

Hordeum distichon

Barley, known to practically everyone as a food of value, is also a remedial agent in that it is a demulcent and indicated in the relief of practically all stomach and intestinal irritations. Due to the large content of sodium in barley, it is of much value in the diet of those sufferng from rheumatism and arthritis by keeping the calcium in solution.

The green sprouts of barley are rich in many mineral elements and with the sprouts of alfalfa offer organic elements essential to health.

Barley, soaked for 8 hours before, added to boiled vegetables should become part of all vegetable soups.

In acidity and inflammation of the mucous membrane of the digestive system, barley water as part of warm milk and beaten egg white gives excellent service. This combination is also indicated in dysentery and diarrhoea. Barley water should be used instead of plain water and mixed with the milk in infant feeding or where there is stomach or intestinal irritation indicated by constant eructions, dysentery, and diarrhoea.

BLACK CURRANT LEAVES

Ribes nigrum

Common name: Quinsy Berry. Squinancy Berry.

The whooping cough remedy. Of much value in various forms of catarrh. Effective as a diuretic.

Generally used as an infusion. One teaspoon of the powdered leaves in a cup of boiling water, steeped for one-half hour, 3 or 4 cups a day. It is well to combine it with other agents for the same conditions.

BLUEBERRIES

Vaccinium Myrtillus

Common names: Bilberry, Whortleberry, Burren Myrtle.

The family diabetic remedy. The Blueberry known throughout many states in America is an astringent. The infusion made with

Blueberry leaves has been a household remedy wherever the Blueberry plant is known. Many diabetic sufferers, who have reached the stage where insulin is necessary, continue to take this infusion.

Unfortunately no cure for the disease has yet been found once the disease has advanced to a condition where insulin is necessary, although the claims of cure are many as a result of taking Blueberry infusion before the disease had advanced to the insulin stage.

In diabetes the diet must be most carefully selected and strictly adhered to. A SINGLE INFRACTION MAY PROVE TO BE FATAL.

The infusion is made by steeping a teaspoon of the leaves in a cup of boiling water for one-half hour, strain, and it is ready to drink, 2 or more cups a day. May be taken with meals instead of coffee or tea.

Dose of tincture 20 to 40 drops.

CAROID

Pawpain

Pawpain, made from the papaya or pawpaw fruit, is an ideal digestive agent in the digestion of proteins, the casein of milk and milk products, and starches. The difference between *Caroid* and *Pepsin* is in the fact that pepsin is active only in an acid field, while *Caroid* acts in almost any field.

Caroid is indicated in all conditions where there is a deficiency of the enzyme.

It is of much value as pretreatment for abscesses, erosions and also ulcers.

Caroid is of much importance where there is a digestive disturbance and an interference with assimilation of food in artificial feeding of infants. It should be mixed with milk or given after feeding with other foods.

COLTSFOOT

Tussilago Farfara

Common names: Coughwort, Foalswort, Horsehoof, Horsefoot, Bull's Foot.

Used in all cases of acute or chronic cough where more or less phlegm is raised. An infusion made of coltsfoot leaves, flowers, and/or roots is generally effective. It is best combined with linden flowers in equal parts.

Whenever there is an indication of physical decline from a known or unknown cause, this tea, infusion, or tincture is of much value.

Coltsfoot, alone or in combination with linden flowers, one-half teaspoon of each steeped in a cup of hot water for one-half hour, drink when cold 3 or more times a day.

The tincture may be used instead of the infusion: dose 15 to 60 drops 3 or more times a day.

COMFREY

Symphytum officinale

A people's remedy for many ailments, Comfrey has long been used as a home or household remedy. In later years the Eclectic School added it to their list of medications, which differed widely from the purposes for which it is now used empirically.

Comfrey is a soothing demulcent, and a gently stimulating tonic to the mucous membrane, especially of the respiratory organs. It is useful in allaying irritations, increasing expectoration and as a tonic for the bronchial tubes. Useful in colds and coughs, it should be combined with other agents such as Wild Cherry, Horehound and Racemosa. In domestic use one ounce of Comfrey was boiled for a few minutes, strained, and either sugar or honey (preferred) added to form a syrup. If to be kept for a period of time, good brandy was added.

It is a possibility that the increasing use and benefit from Comfrey is that it is very rich in easily assimilated organic calcium.

Next to Lobelia, Comfrey is one of the most controversial of all healing agents. Unofficially, it has long been accepted as of great value as a soothing demulcent, a gentle stimulant to the mucous membrane, to allay irritation of the respiratory organs and increase expectoration, and a tonic to the bronchial tubes. It is useful in colds and coughs, especially if combined in an infusion with baked onion juice, sweetened with honey, and taken as warm as possible.

These virtues are generally granted it by all Natura and many physicians of the various schools. To its converts, and there are thousands of them, it is a miracle plant. The relief it has brought in various instances are well authenticated. One thing is certain, it is harmless, and in many instances in which it has brought relief, it was taken or used as a last resource.

Of late years the agent has become respectable, and a reason found for its generally accepted virtue by physicians and laity who have used it or prescribed it is due in part to the discovery that it contains an active principle known as *Allantoin.*

Its proponents or converts become so by what it has done for them. In chronic sores of various types, a poultice made of either the crushed green plant or the powder of the plant has effected elimination of the sores within a short period of time in which all other agents and procedures had failed.

In general Natura practice, Comfrey has been successfully used in ailments diagnosed as arthritis, gall stones, stomach conditions, asthma, and other diametrically different conditions.

These are numerous uncontradicted reports of lung cancer cured where all other means had failed and in which the sole treatment consisted of infusions made from the whole green plant and, even in some instances, of infusion made from the powder of the entire plant.

There are reports of acute cases of ulcerated tonsils with a high temperature present in which infusions of the green plant given frequently—poultices of the dry powder placed about the throat—responded to the treatment within a short period of time.

The infusion has been given successfully in severe liver and stomach conditions in which other forms of treatment reportedly failed.

Comfrey either in the tincture or infusion is given for the purpose of cleansing the entire system of impurities and establishing a normal condition.

The dosage of the tincture is 5 to 20 drops 4 times a day. Infusion is made out of either the entire fresh plant or the powder of the entire plant, 1 teaspoon steeped in a cup of hot water for one-half hour, stir frequently, take 4 times a day.

Although Comfrey, as a remedial agent, is highly controversial, those who have suffered from ailments (wholly different in nature which had resisted all manner of treatment) are legion and these are firmly convinced of its virtue even in the case of various forms of cancer.

DANDELION

Leontodon taraxacum

Common names: Blow Ball, Cankerwort.

Dandelion root is essentially a household remedy. It is a stomach tonic possessing slightly diuretic and aperient action.

Dandelion has a beneficial influence upon the biliary organs, removing torpor and engorgement of the liver as well as of the spleen, and will do best when combined with *Hydrastis* and *Chionanthus*.

It is of benefit in dropsy when due to inertia of the abdominal organs and also in uterine obstructions. In chronic skin diseases it is always indicated.

Dandelion root cut up and dried is used for coffee by innumerable people. From a health point of view, it is a more desirable drink than coffee or tea. For this purpose it is frequently combined with roasted acorns and roasted rye in equal parts, or according to taste. As a vegetable for salads, it has no equal being rich in many minerals. It is a medical-vegetable plant.

Dose tincture: 5 to 40 drops.

For infusion, fill a cup with the green leaves, add boiling water, steep one-half hour or longer. Drink when cold, 3 or 4 times a day. Or add a teaspoon of the cut or powdered root to a cup of boiling water, and steep one-half hour. Drink when cold, 3 times a day.

DWARF ELDER

Sambucus Ebulus

Common names: Wild Elder, Danewort, Walewort.

Dwarf Elder was long considered and used in the treatment of dropsy. It was also used—and still is—for abdominal disturbances, and it is considered effective in the elimination of effete material through the kidneys.

Infusion is made by steeping a teaspoon of powdered root in a cup of hot water for one-half hour, divide into 3 doses, one portion every 4 hours.

The tincture of Dwarf Elder may be substituted for the infusion. Dose 3 to 15 drops.

An ointment, made with either the infusion or tincture and melted lard, has long been a family remedy for burns and scalding.

EYEBRIGHT

Euphrasia officinalis

Common name: Eyebright (Euphrasia).

The inflamed eye remedy. To be used in combination with fennel. An infusion of 1 teaspoon of Eyebright in a cup of boiling water, steep one-half hour, strain carefully, and use for eye wash. Cold compresses of eyebright may be used to cover the eyes.

Infusion of Eyebright, made in same manner, is frequently used in nasal congestion, catarrh, cough, hoarseness, and earache and headache associated with a cold. The infusion for this purpose is made in the manner stated.

The tincture, 15 to 40 drops every 3 to 4 hours, may be used instead of the infusion.

FENNEL

Foeniculum vulgare

Common names: Wild Fennel, Sweet Fennel, Large Fennel.

Called the wind colic remedy—mother's friend. No agent has proven so effective and reliable in a mother's hand for the relief for wind colic in babies as fennel.

To use, the seed may be bought and kept on reserve for instant use. One teaspoon is added to a cup of milk and boiled slowly for a few minutes, strain, and let cool, then drink. In severe attacks an infusion may be made of the seed, and a compress placed over the stomach.

The seed of Fennel made into an infusion has long been used as an eyewash. For this purpose it is best combined with Eyebright and eyes washed with it 3 or 4 times a day.

Dosage of Fennel, 10 to 30 or more drops in warm water according to age as required.

FLAXSEED (LINSEED)
Linum usitatissimum

Flaxseed is too well-known for too long a time to need description. It is the *ideal* base for all poultices and compresses when applied as hot as the patient can bear it. Keep warm with hot water bottle or electric pad. Any form of herbal medication may be combined with it.

GINGER
Zingiber officinale

Zingiber is an almost universal agent, almost too well-known to require description. It is a domestic or household remedy.

It is excellent for children's colics and cramps, and expelling gas. It is of much value in the beginning of colds by quickly sending the blood to the surface. Its prompt use will frequently avert pneumonia and other serious developing maladies.

A pleasant and almost universal way to prepare it is to mix thoroughly one-half teaspoon of pulverized ginger with a teaspoon or more of honey, pouring over it a cup of boiling water. Adults prefer to add an ounce or more of good brandy or other liquor and retire. If tincture is used, 15 or more drops (warm) depending on age.

In the onset of pneumonia or pleurisy a combination of:

Tincture of Ginger (*Zingiber officinale*)	10 to 40 drops
Tincture of Pleurisy Root (*Ascleptias tuberosa*)	10 to 20 drops
Tincture of Cayenne Pepper (*Capsicum frutescens*)	2 to 3 drops

In hot water, depending on age and condition, every 3 to 4 hours.

Zingiber may be used as the base to almost every other agent in the onset of chills and cold. In earlier days, and even today in remote places where the services of a physician are not easily obtained, families prepare a syrup of Ginger by adding 6 drams of the tincture to a pint of simple syrup in readiness for the onset of chills or colds by members of the family, or by having the Thomsonian preparations in the medicine closet.

HEMLOCK CONIUM MACULATUM

Abies canadensis

Common names: Hemlock spruce, Pinus bark.

Hemlock is an astringent, stimulant, and antiseptic. It has long been used in the treatment of simple inflammation, skin afflictions, and ulcerations.

Abies alone or combined with other agents for the treatment of rhinitis, pharyngitis when tenacious mucus secretions are present, and usually effective in tonsilitis.

The infusion or tincture of Hemlock is very helpful when used as a douche or on tampons in the treatment of vaginitis, leucorrhea, and cervical erosions.

Infusion is made by adding 3 tablespoons of the leaves to 6 ounces of boiling water, steep one-half hour, strain, 1 teaspoon every 2 or 3 hours.

Dose of tincture, 5 to 10 drops. Hemlock should be used *with much caution.*

Hemlock is one of the most important ingredients in the original Thomsonian No. 3 and is best used in that manner when its use is indicated.

JUNIPER BERRIES

Juniperus communis

Juniper Berries, generally in infusion, has long been a family remedy as a diuretic. It is indicated when there is irritation of the urinary passage or when the kidneys do not function properly.

It was—and still is—much employed in dropsical conditions where it is best used in small doses. Small doses reduce irritation, while large doses may increase it. It is counter-indicated in neuritis.

To make an infusion, the berries are generally prepared by macerating (softening by soaking) several tablespoons of the berries, then adding them to a pint of boiling water for one-half hour or more, cool, and this is divided into four portions, taken morning, noon, afternoon, and evening.

Dose of the tincture 10 to 30 drops.

KNOTGRASS

Polyganum aviculare

Common names: Beggarweed, Pigweed, Red Robin. Better known as Wiregrass, the curse of gardeners.

It has been and still is used as an astringent and diuretic, but more especially as a gravel remedy.

Its main influence is on the bladder not only to help remove small stones but to prevent their formation. The family use was mostly for this purpose. In making an infusion it is best combined with Shave Grass, also a gravel remedy, in equal parts.

To make an infusion, add a teaspoon of Knotgrass into a cup of boiling water, steep one-half hour. When cold, take 1 cup 2 or 3 times a day. If Shave Grass is added, use 1 teaspoon of each in a pint of water, divide into two portions.

Dose of tincture of Knotgrass, or combination, 15 to 30 drops in plenty of water 3 or more times a day.

LINDEN FLOWERS

Tilia Europaea

Common name: Lime Tree, Common Lime.

The chronic cough remedy. An infusion made of Linden Flower leaves will help remove mucus from the lungs and trachea, and prove of much value in bronchial catarrh. For this purpose it is best combined with Coltsfoot.

The infusion will also flush the kidneys of mucus when present and avoid the development of serious abdominal conditions.

The infusion is made with 1 teaspoon of the leaves in hot water, steep one-half hour, permit to cool, and drink. This may be done as frequently as necessary.

Tilia may be given in the tincture; 15 to 40 drops as indicated by conditions.

MAYFLOWER

Pulsatilla Nigricans

The woman's remedy and the Neurasthenic's remedy.

Pulsatilla is an ideal agent in all complaints having their origin in an abnormal, abused or unbalanced generative system. Its indications are varied: fear of impending dangers, unrest, looking on the dark side of everything, melancholia, gastric disturbances, morning sickness, and eructions after eating, flatulent colic, and abnormalities of menstrual period, including pain in the small of the back. Best given only in the tincture, 1 to 2 drops, 3 times a day. MUST BE TAKEN CAUTIOUSLY. WHEN POSSIBLE, UNDER THE SUPERVISION OF A PHYSICIAN.

Pulsatilla may be truthfully called the neurotic remedy. The *Natura* physician would not practice without it.

MILKWORT

Polygala vulgaris

Common name: Rogation Flower, Gang Flower.

The milk or lactation remedy. Milkwort is generally used in conjunction with *Mitchella*. Women approaching motherhood who have the normal desire to suckle their child, and who want to be certain they have sufficient milk for the purpose; or who find their milk supply diminishing should make an infusion of a combination of Squaw Vine and Milkwort, a teaspoon of each added to a pint of hot water, steeped for 30 minutes, cool. A tablespoon every few hours. Today the tincture is more desirable, 9 or more drops of *Polygala* every 4 hours, or 15 drops of the combined tinctures.

MULLEIN, GREAT

Verbascum thapsus

Common names: Velvet Dock, Velvet Plant, Flannel Leaf.

Verbascum is a demulcent, diuretic, anodyne, and antispasmodic. It is a winter remedy and is much used in affections of the throat, catarrh, mucus on the chest, and shortness of breath.

In earlier times, the dried flowers were boiled in milk (a tablespoon of the powdered flowers to a pint of milk), cooled and a tablespoon taken every few hours, or as necessary. It is made now generally with boiling water instead of milk.

For colds in the chest, make a compress by boiling the flowers in vinegar for 15 minutes, adding 8 to 12 drops to the infusion, placing it over the chest and keeping it warm by a hot water bottle or an electric pad, changing every 3 to 5 hours.

Dosage of the tincture, 15 to 40 drops in warm water every 2 to 4 hours according to condition.

A very early German remedy used in deafness as a result of dried ear wax, wax too soft or insufficient, is Mullein oil, sun distilled from green Mullein flowers, 3 to 5 drops twice a day, until the condition is corrected.

OAK BARK

Quercus robur

Common name: Tanner's Bark. Although the white oak bark made into an infusion was best known as a goitre remedy, it was (still is) used more often in ailments of the stomach, the elimination of mucus, general dyspepsia, normalization of the liver and spleen, and as a diuretic.

The infusion is made by steeping a tablespoon of the powdered bark in a pint of hot water for one-half hour, let cool and strain. Dose: 1 or 2 ounces every few hours. Tincture: 5 to 10 drops every four hours *to be taken with caution*. In general practice, it is usually combined with thyroid and other agents.

For other conditions, a tablespoon of the infusion is taken between each meal, or a coffee made of the roasted acorns with meals.

OATS AND OAT BEARDS

Avena sativa

Common names: Groat. One of the best natural tonics long used as a family remedy is an infusion made with oat beards, or in its place the tincture of oats. So general was this opinion of oats that it gave rise to the expression "he is feeling his oats" when speaking of a spirited horse who had been fed oats.

Avena sativa, as well as the tea made from the oat beards, has long been recognized by people as a naturalizer to the sexual system.

The tea is made by steeping a teaspoon of the beards in a cup of hot water, for 5 or more minutes, strain, and if desired add cream and a sweetener (sugar or honey) and drink with meals. An infusion made in the same way but steeped for a longer time may be taken 3 times a day.

A tea or infusion long used by women to retain their youth after their thirty-fifth birthday was made into a coffee-like drink by combining oat beards, roasted acorns, and chicory, in equal proportions, and drunk with their meals instead of tea or coffee.

Dose of the tincture, *Avena Saliva,* 10 to 20 drops, 3 times a day.

ONION

Allium cepa

The lowly pungent onion, possibly the most used in former times of all family remedies, is still much used in country districts and even in cities by mothers who were taught its virtues in their childhood.

The onion is a stimulant, diuretic, and expectorant, and it is extremely useful in colds, coughs, and croup in children; and when properly prepared, also in colds and coughs in older people.

In former times when wood and coal stoves were in use, onions were placed in the compartment of the stove which led from the fireplace to the chimney. They were left there until thoroughly soft, then mashed so the juice could easily be squeezed out of it. Honey was added to this onion juice, and given in teaspoon doses every one-half hour or oftener as necessary.

In cases where there is an indication that the lungs might be affected, a poultice of baked onions should be placed over the lungs and kept warm by means of a hot water bottle or electric pad.

Onions may be baked in the oven though they do not appear to be as effective in releasing the valuable juice as was the former means.

Any other medication may be combined with the onion juice but is best given between the juice doses.

Many parents in country distrcts believe this onion-honey treatment more effective and dependable than any medical treatment.

PENNYROYAL, AMERICAN

Mentha pulegium

Common names: Tickweed, Squawweed.

An age-old domestic family remedy, formerly known to almost every woman, was gathered when in bloom, dried and kept for use until the next gathering.

Pennyroyal is an aromatic, stimulating, and relaxing diaphoretic, most pleasant to taste. In hot infusion or tincture in hot water, it has always been popular as a remedy for breaking up colds readily, and can be freely given to children of all ages. It is also a remedy for the menstrual flow when it is retarded by congestion or colds. Although a diaphoretic it is also an antispasmodic nervine and often found of much value in dysmenorrhoea in nervous women and in hysteria.

In hot infusion or tincture in hot water, it is a valuable agent in the eruptive diseases of children and can be freely given.

The hot infusion or tincture in hot water is an excellent agent in colic, flatulence, restlessness, and peevishness in children, as well as in nervousness and feverishness in childhood complaints. Whenever there is either a cold or a temperature, it should be freely given as an agent with which to combine other and stronger agents, especially such as Pleurisy Root and Scullcap.

Locally, Pennroyal has long been used in hot fomentation to relieve congestions, mixed with *Lobelia* or other agents, whether of heart, lungs, stomach, uterus, bladder, or kidneys.

The tea or infusion may be given freely; it being non-poisonous and non-toxic. Dose of tincture, 20 to 60 drops as indicated. For children it is best given in small doses in hot water frequently.

PRICKLY ASH

Xanthoxylum Americanum

Prickly Ash is of the nature of *Capsicum.* Where continued effects are desired, a small amount of *Capsicum* should be added to it.

The bark, the leaves, and the berries are of almost equal potency, although the leaves lend themselves more readily to infusions.

Prickly Ash is a splendid innocent agent in stomach disorders, particularly indicated where digestion is slow, permitting fermentation and the formation of gas. Where the tincture is not to be obtained, infusions taken warm are effective. Effectiveness may be increased by the addition of *Hydrastis* and *Capsicum* best given shortly before meals.

In most cases of illness where there is a deficiency of secretions, dryness of mouth and feces, uterine cramps, and colic, Prickly Ash is a splendid agent.

In chronic cases it may be used where there is lack of hepatic and pancreatic activity, chronic muscular rheumatism, lumbago, scrofula, and temporary paralysis.

In acute conditions, it gives best results in warm infusions, one-half teaspoon of the powdered leaves or bark steeped one-half hour in hot water and strained, take every 3 hours.

In chronic digestive intestinal conditions the infusion or the tincture may be given, *Zanthoxylum,* in doses of 5 to 10 drops: in combination, 3 drops of *Hydrastis* and 1 drop of *Capsicum,* always in warm water for quick action.

In syphilis, scrofula, and like ailments, the tincture is more desirable than the infusion, 15 drops with the addition of *Pytholacca,* 5 drops.

In rheumatism, arthritis, paralysis, and like ailments, 20 drops of the tincture with the addition of 5 drops of tincture of *Pytholacca* is indicated.

The greatest usefulness of Prickly Ash is in atonic stomach and intestinal conditions and is combined with *Hydrastis* and *Capsicum.*

PRIMROSE

Primula vulgaris

Common names: Butter Rose, English Cowslip.

This is almost a legendary remedy in the treatment of articular rheumatism, first used—and still much used—as an infusion and later in tincture form. The infusion appears to be more effective. For best results, an equal portion of Motherwort is combined with Primrose.

This is prepared by adding a teaspoon of each to a pint of water, boil slowly to half the amount. Cool, strain, divide into three portions—one portion before each meal. This combination is of much benefit also for headaches due to a stomach condition. The preparation MUST be made fresh daily. This is actually best with all infusions unless alcohol is added, or made into a syrup.

Dosage of tincture, 5 to 20 drops, 3 or 4 times a day depending on condition.

ROSEMARY

Rosemarinus officinalis

Freely used in all instances where there is a torpid condition of the liver and a predisposition toward dropsy. It is equally indicated in all conditions where there is congestion of the system with morbid matter, as indicated by frequent colds.

Rosemary tea, best combined with Sassafras root, has long been used as the ideal fall and spring cleaner in place of the age-old sulphur and molasses combination.

Infusion of either, or both in combination, is best for the purpose: 1 teaspoon each steeped in a cup of boiling water for one-half hour, 1 tablespoon divided into 3 parts.

Dose of the tincture of Rosemary, 10 to 20 drops. Of the combination of Rosemary and Sassafras, 14 to 30 drops in water 3 times a day for a month as a systemic cleanser.

SAGE

Salvia officinala

The night-sweat remedy. Sage is a natural astringent and may be freely used without danger. In fevers it should be given in cold infusions as a substitute for the fruit juices now so generally given.

Salvia is of much value in liver and kidney conditions, but it is best combined with Rosemary and Motherwort: An infusion is made of 2 tablespoons Sage; 1 tablespoon Rosemary *Rosenarinus*, one-half tablespoonful of Motherwort *Leonurus*. Steep in 1 pint of water for one-half hour, and strain. Dose: 1 teaspoon before meals.

In stomach complaints combine 2 parts Sage with one-fourth part Goldenseal and one-half part of Yellow Gentian. Two ounces of this mixture should be steeped in a pint of water for one-half hour. Dose: 1 tablespoon before meals.

Sage used alone for night sweats is best made into an infusion. Use two teaspoons in a pint of boiling water, steep an hour, drain, and when cold, take 1 tablespoon every hour or two until sweats are overcome. Any medication for fever may be combined with it.

Dosage: Tincture of Sage, 15 to 40 drops, 3 or 4 times a day.

ST. JOHN'S WORT

Hypericum perforatum

The family remedy to overcome bedwetting. For this purpose a tea is made with one-half teaspoon of leaves and flowers of the herb steeped for an hour and taken regularly each evening before retiring.

St. John's Wort picked when in full bloom and used either fresh or dried as a tea or infusion was a favorite remedy for stomach ailments. Especially for the fathers of the family! They placed a goodly portion of the herb in a quart bottle, filled it with whiskey, and set it aside for use. One tablespoon as required. Yellow Gentian, one part to every four parts of St. John's Wort was added to either tea or whiskey, when taken as a liver corrector.

SILVERWEED

Potentilla anserina

Common names: Silvery Cinquefoil, Cramp Weed, Goose Tansy, Moot Grass.

Tetanus is a dangerous condition, and there is need for the immediate services of a physician. However, throughout time including the present, where in outlying rural districts, it is impossible to secure the services of a physician when there is an immediate need. Under these circumstances many families stored a supply of *Silverweed* for emergency need.

A teaspoon of the powdered weed is boiled, either in water or milk (10 minutes in water, less in milk), and this given every hour or oftener in combination with 10 or more drops of *Lobelia*. In conjunction, the body should be immersed in water as hot as can be borne until it relaxes. The wound should be cauterized and kept clean by the frequent use of strong undiluted antiseptics.

Dosage of tincture: 15 to 40 drops in water every 1 or 2 hours.

STRAWBERRY LEAVES

Frageria vesca
Fragaria americana

The Eczema remedy. The medicinal content in Strawberry Leaves is an excellent blood purifier; and their special influence has always been considered by users of Nature's remedies as possessing special effectiveness on that class of bodily poisons which causes a chronic or acute irritation of the skin and is generally known as *Eczema*.

To be most effective it should be combined with equal parts of Dandelion (*Taraxacum*) and Burdock, and just enough Rhubarb (*Rheum*) to assure regular bowel evacuation.

The infusion is made with 1 teaspoon each of Strawberry Leaves and Dandelion root and one-half teaspoon of Rhubarb and Burdock steeped in a pint of hot water for one-half hour; strain, and when cold add small amount of brandy to prevent fermentation. Dose:

1 tablespoon 3 or 4 times a day. If the Rhubarb content acts too drastically, the amount is to be reduced.

Dosage of the tincture *Fragaria,* 5 to 15 drops in water 3 times a day.

SUMACH

Rhus Glabra
Rhus Blabrum

Common names: Smooth Sumach, Scarlet Sumach.

Sumach is rather a family or domestic remedy than a physician's agent. It is still used extensively in country districts and requests for instructions for its preparation and use are frequent.

Sumach is a composite agent. The berries are diuretic, the bark is astringent and antiseptic.

It is a splendid agent, a demulcent, in all conditions where the mucous membranes are in an irritated condition as in dysentery, as well as when the urine is scalding the urinary passage.

The bark is a most stimulating astringent and toning agent, valuable in leucorrhoea, rectal conditions, chronic diarrhea, and rectal hemorrhages. In inflammation of the bladder the fresh leaves or berries are best used in an infusion, and will usually give prompt relief. *Sumach* is frequently used in scrofula.

The leaves and bark are best made into an infusion, a teaspoon of either or one-half portion of each in a cup of boiling water. Steep half an hour; when cold take 2 or more cups a day.

A syrup may be made with the berries by covering them with boiling water, steep for an hour, strain and add honey, boil into a syrup, and bottle for future use.

The infusion is much used in combination with Blueberry leaves (equal parts) in diabetes.

For summer diarrhea and dysentery, Blackberry (equal parts) should be added in making the syrup.

The syrup may also be made from the bark and fresh leaves. Instead of honey, a sufficient amount of good brandy is added to prevent it from fermenting. However, the infusion is best for quick results. In acute cases the syrup should be taken in hot water.

Dose of tincture, 10 to 20 drops.

SWEET FLAG

Acorus Calamus

Common names: Myrtle Flag, Sweet Grass, Calamus, Sweet Sedge.

The ancient water-brash (watery eruction) remedy. When everything tried fails to stop the eruction of the burning water from the stomach into the throat, *Calamus* will generally do it. Those suffering from this condition should collect the root during the summer or fall, cut it into small pieces and dry (or obtain it from herb house) to have on hand when required. A small piece chewed and the juice swallowed will offer prompt relief. In many instances those suffering from stomach discomfort from some unknown reason will find *Calamus* a remedy by chewing it several times a day. Where attacks of waterbrash are frequent, tincture *Hydrastis*, Golden Seal, 5 to 10 drops in water should be taken in addition before meals.

Children suffering continually from gas in the stomach should be given a weak tea of it at regular intervals. It is an innocent, effective remedy.

Sweet Flag is of great help in the treatment of scrofula—a legendary disease dating from the time of the Egyptians—and should be included with other agents for the treatment of this condition.

Dosage: Tincture of *Calamus,* 10 to 40 drops in water according to age and severity of condition.

TANSY

Tanacetum vulgare

Common names: Arbor Vitae, Yellow Cedar.

Tansy was once a household remedy possessed of virtue as well as a vice (if an herb may be thought of as possessing a vice). Many have thought of it only as a means to cause abortion. *It is certain that pregnant women should not use it.* It is also an irritant and narcotic, and in improper dosage is to be avoided and condemned.

Tansy is an extremely bitter tonic. A weak tea made of the herb or small doses of the tincture is excellent for hysteria and also in the relief of the suppression of menses due to causes other than pregnancy.

It has been much used as a family medicine and by *Natura* physicians to strengthen weak veins and kidneys, and is of benefit in strangury. When given as a cold infusion, it is a tonic and an aid to digestion.

Tansy had—and still has—a place in the family medicine chest when it is difficult to obtain the services of a physician.

Dose of the tincture is from 5 to 10 drops; the larger dose only in extreme cases of hysteria and suppression of the menses due to causes other than pregnancy.

Although considered a "family" medicine, *it is best taken only under the care of a physician or in emergencies.*

Infusion: One teaspoon of Tansy steeped in a pint of boiling water for one-half hour; one teaspoon every 3 hours.

TORMENTIL
Potentilla Tormentilla

The roots of *Tormentilla* are a mild stimulating astringent. It favorably influences the alvine mucous membrane and is of benefit in ordinary diarrhoea and mild hemorrhages. In domestic medicine it is chiefly known as a sex remedy. Like Scurvy Grass it was employed by the country people as a remedy in acute sex diseases such as gonorrhoea. It is used in the same manner as Scurvy Grass or in combination with it. Today there are much more effective remedies for this disease.

It is still much used, and effectively, by women as a douche for the "whites" *(fluor albus),* because it is a natural cleanser. An infusion is made by steeping a tablespoon in a quart of water for 30 or more minutes; strain, and use while still slightly warm.

VERVAIN, EUROPEAN
Verbena officinalis

Vervain has long been used as a family whooping cough remedy. The roots of vervain are combined with Violet Bloom (often called

Bittersweet) in equal parts, and 1 teaspoon of the mixture steeped in a pint of boiling water for 30 minutes, strained, and a teaspoon given frequently to control the spasms. Elimination must be kept free.

Dosage of tincture Vervain, 20 to 40 drops in water as frequently as necessary.

SWEET VIOLET

Violet odorata

Like Vervain root the leaves of the fragrant Violet have an effective influence on controlling whooping cough as well as other coughs, especially when accompanied with shortness of breath. It is well combined with Vervain root in equal parts for an infusion, 1 tablespoon of the mixture steeped in a pint of boiling water, strained, and one tablespoon taken frequently.

Coltsfoot, Vervain, and Violet in equal part, may also be combined for an infusion and given in the same manner.

WATERCRESS

Nasturtium officinale

Watercress as an infusion was long used as an effective blood purifier and given frequently. Since it has become elevated to a delicious and desirable vegetable or garnish, it is best used by eating the fresh Watercress. For this purpose it must be eaten regularly as a salad once a day.

YELLOW CEDAR

Thuja occidentalis

Common names: Arbor Vitae, Thuja.

This is a remedy for muscular aches and pains not due to arthritis or rheumatism.

Yellow Cedar is useful in chronic and subacute prostatic conditions where immediate operation is not indicated; for incontinence of urine, spermatorrhoea, gonorrhoea, vesical atony, and like ailments. The dosage is small, 3 to 10 drops; the tincture must be made from the green herb.

Yellow Cedar ointment is often successfully applied to warts, Also as an application to fistulae, bleeding moles, soft chancres, fissures, urethral carbuncles, and various indolent lesions. The non-alcoholic tincture is best used for external application.

In muscular pains, the tincture should be taken internally and the salve applied externally.

Three grain tablets of Yellow Cedar are much used by those who do not desire or who fear the contamination of their blood by serums made from animal pus. Use 3 times a day for 3 months prior to inoculations, and continue for 3 months thereafter.

10.

OTHER NATURAL AGENTS LONG USED IN HOUSEHOLD OR DOMESTIC PRACTICE

AGRIMONY

Agrimonia Eupatoria

Common names: Cockleburr, Sticklewort.

Agrimony has long been used in domestic practice for bedwetting and weakness of the bladder. It was also much used for loose coughs and sore mouths.

The entire herb and/or dry root is made into an infusion, 1 ounce to the pint of boiling water, given in tablespoon doses every 3 hours; or in 2 tablespoon doses every 4 hours, and again in a very small amount of water just before retiring.

ALFALFA

Medicago sativa

Common name: Lucerne, Alfalfa Buffalo Herb.

A tonic and nutrient long recognized as rich in vitamins and minerals. It may be freely used where vitality is low, as a tea with, or between, meals. Alfalfa tea is delightful with meals. It is of much value where vitality is low due to any cause.

ALLSPICE

Pimento officinalis

Common names: Pimento, Jamaica Pepper.

Allspice should not be used or given to anyone suffering with any form of stomach complaint.

143

Allspice is a common household spice frequently used in the preparation of food. It is of much benefit in ordinary diarrhoea. It is made more effective by adding a small amount of cloves.

Allspice is a mild astringent. In cholera infantum it is of much benefit; it relieves colic due to colds.

While Allspice may be given as the tincture, it is best used as an infusion made by steeping a teaspoon of it in boiling water for 30 minutes, strain. Dose: a teaspoon in water every hour or oftener according to condition.

AMERICAN CENTAURY

Sabatia angularis

Common names: Rose Pink, Bitterbloom, Bittle Clover.

The convalescence remedy. *Sabbatia* is an excellent bitter tonic. It is often used either alone or with other tonics such as oats. It is indicated in simple forms of dyspepsia, and may be added to other agents for that purpose. Infusion is made by adding a teaspoon of the cut or powdered herb in a cup of boiling water, steep for one-half hour, take a tablespoon every few hours. It is frequently made by adding 4 teaspoons into a pint of good whisky or brandy, take a tablespoon every 3 hours.

Dose of the tincture in water: 15 to 40 drops every 3 or 4 hours.

AMERICAN SENNA (WILD)

Cassia Marilandica

Common names: Wild Senna, Locust Plant.

The household cathartic. Although universally used as an infusion or tea for constipation, it is too harsh to be used alone and should be combined with other agents such as *Cascara Sagrada,* Rhubarb, and agents that will fortify it, but reduce its harshness. *Senna* preparations properly combined may be readily obtained and best used instead of the infusion.

ANISE

Pimpinella anisum

Anise is a pleasant stimulating aromatic, and it is very acceptable to children. It has long been a household remedy in colic and flatulence in children. It is best given in doses of 1 or 2 drops on lumps of sugar. Being non-poisonous, it may be given as frequently as necessary.

Parents frequently give their children cakes covered with Anise seed during the holiday season to overcome incidence of the overeating of sweets.

ASPARAGUS

Asparagus officinalis

Common name: Sparrow Grass.

Asparagus is a diaphoretic, aperient, and an important agent in many health preparations. Its chief use is in combination with other more harsh remedies for costiveness. It combines well with *Cascara Sagrada,* Senna, and other herbal agents. Best when consumed fresh as a vegetable.

BALM

Melissa officinalis

Common names: Lemon Balm, Garden Balm, Sweet Balm.

Balm belongs to the mint family and may be used as mint teas generally are. It is a diaphoretic and in warm infusion will help to produce sweating when wanted in fevers. It is frequently so employed in teas to which lemon juice is added, supplying the now much acclaimed Vitamin C.

Infusion is made by adding 4 teaspoons of the herb to a pint of boiling water; steep one-half an hour, strain. A tablespoon or 2 to a cup of hot water, taking as frequently as desired, or, in cases where sweating is desired, until there is a free perspiration.

BALM OF GILEAD
Populus balsamifera

Populus is a stimulating expectorant, and beneficially is included in cough syrup. It is useful in coughs of long standing where the lungs are feeble and unable to throw off accumulations in the air passages, but must *not* be used in irritation of the lungs.

Populus is best used in the tincture. An infusion cannot be made of it because of its resinous nature.

One-half ounce of the buds soaked in alcohol added to any cough syrup will serve well.

Dosage of tincture, 5 to 20 drops in water according to age and seriousness of cough.

BEARBERRY
Arctostaphylos Uva-Ursi

Common names: Upland Cranberry, Arberry.

Bearberry is an astringent and tonic and especially indicated where a dependable diuretic is required.

Contrary to most herbals, it is not best given in infusions, but by immersing the leaves in either alcohol or a good brandy, and taking a teaspoon of this preparation in a cup of hot or cold water, depending on results desired, 2 or more times a day.

Dose of tincture to be given in the same manner and generally more certain. Dosage: 10 to 25 drops in water, 3 or more times a day according to symptoms.

BITTERSWEET
Solanum Dulcamara

Common names: Mortal, Woody Nightshade, Felon Wort, Fever Twig, Violet Bloom, Scarletberry.

Bittersweet has been considered a mild narcotic because of its relaxant influence. Its influence, when taken internally, is chiefly upon the glandular system. It is best combined with *Queen's Root* and Yellow Dock in an infusion, 1 teaspoon of each in a pint of boiling water, steep one-half hour, take 1 teaspoon or more in a cup of warm water as required. May be given in tincture, dosage: 10 to 15 drops, 3 or 4 times a day.

One pound of the cut bark of Bittersweet *slowly* heated in a pound of lard for 8 hours forms a splendid ointment to apply to irritable skin conditions, piles, burns, scalds, and other skin diseases.

BLACKBERRY, AMERICAN
Rubus villosus

Common names: Bramble, Gout Berry, Cloud Berry, Dewberry.

Blackberry or Dewberry root is too well known to require description, for its usage as an astringent and tonic in almost all forms of diarrhoea, especially of children during the summer months.

Infusion is made by steeping a teaspoon of the cut root or leaves, or combination of both, in a cup of boiling water for one-half hour. Given cold in tablespoon doses as frequently as necessary.

Dose of tincture: 15 to 40 drops in water according to age, as frequently as necessary.

BLACK ROOT
Leptandra Virginica

Common names: Culver's Physic, Tall Speedwell, Tall Veronica, Culver's Root.

Liver or bile remedy. Black Root is a relaxant, exerting its action on the liver and is mostly used as a physic when a free flow of bile is essential. It is also a tonic. In torpidity of the liver, especially when headache is associated with it, Black Root is an ideal agent.

An infusion is made by steeping a teaspoon of the cut or powdered root in a cup of boiling water for 30 minutes. Divide into 3 portions taking 1 part before each meal.

Black Root is best taken as a tincture. Dose: 2 to 4 drops in water. Whether it is taken as an infusion or tincture, it is generally slow in action.

Black Root combines well with other agents directly influencing the action of the liver.

BLOODROOT

Sanguinaria canadensis

Common names: Red Puccoon, Indian Plant, Tetterwort.

Sanguinaria is a most valuable remedy in the hands of the skilled *Natura* physician. *To be taken only in small doses as it is poisonous. Never* desirable in large doses.

It is an effective remedy in acute and chronic rhinitis where there is an offensive discharge and irritating cough with difficult respiration. *Sanguinaria* is valuable in all respiratory diseases, especially in affections of the nose, pharynx, fauces, larynx, and bronchi in which there is a deficiency in the mucous membrane indicated by a dry throat and a dry irritating cough.

Dose: Tincture, 5 to 20 drops according to symptoms. *To be taken only in an emergency or under the care of a physician. Poisonous.*

BLUE COHOSH

Caulophyllum thalictroides

Common name: Papoose Root.

The woman's remedy. The Indians used this herb as an agent for the relief of colic and cramps in children (hence the name "papoose root"), and cramps during menstruation, frequently combined with Black Cohosh for this purpose.

It is an agent now chiefly given for menstrual difficulties, promoting freer flow and affording relief from the usual pain associated with this condition. It is much used also in promoting labor pains.

An infusion is made by steeping an ounce of the cut or powdered root in a pint of boiling water for one-half hour, given in hot water,

2 tablespoons every 2 or 3 hours. In spasms it may be given with hot water more frequently.

Dosage of tincture: 5 to 10 drops.

BROOM

Cytisus scoparius

Common names: Link, Genista, Banal.

This kidney remedy for scanty urine has been long used and of great benefit in many cases. The tops of the plant are used for infusion. One teaspoon steeped in boiling water for one-half hour, let cool, 1 or more cups a day, according to need.

Tincture: 20 to 40 drops 2 or 3 times a day.

Dandelion *(Taraxacum),* in equal part, is frequently combined with Broom for Cystitis.

BRYONY, EUROPEAN WHITE

Bryonia alba

Common names: Wild Bryony, White Bryony.

A remedy in the relief of the spasms of whooping cough. Best used as a tincture, dose: 5 to 10 drops. Except in an emergency, *use only under the care of a physician as it is poisonous.*

BUCKHORNE DRAKE

Osmunda regalis

Common names: Male Fern, King's Fern, Royal Flowering Fern.

A tonic and styptic much used in coughs associated with, or following, a cold. Valuable in diarrhoea and convalescence.

Infusion: cut roots or powder, steep 1 teaspoon in a cup of boiling water for 30 minutes, take 1 tablespoon every hour, or as required. Tincture: 20 to 40 drops.

BUGLEWEED

Lycopus Virginicus

Common names: Water Bugle, Gypsy Wort.

A soothing astringent acting as a nervine. It is indicated in loose coughs and hemorrhages from lungs and bladder and in incontinence of urine.

Infusion: One ounce of the herb steeped in a pint of boiling water for one-half hour, take 2 or 3 tablespoons every 2 hours. Dose of tincture: 20 to 40 drops.

Lycopus has been much used in the treatment of fistula, applied to the affected part until granulation is established.

BUTTERNUT

Juglans cinerea

Common names: Clotburr, Bardana, White Walnut.

Juglans' chief influence is upon the lower bowels, and for this purpose it is unexcelled in prolapsus and constipation due to sluggishness of the large bowel. It is best administered as a syrup by boiling a pound of the bark in water and then evaporating it to one pint, adding a pound of sugar and turning it into a syrup. Dose: One tablespoon. When a quick cathartic is desired, Senna may be added. Juglans in small amounts is an agent valuable in protracted febrile diseases.

Dosage tincture of Butternut 1 to 15 drops 3 times a day according to condition.

CALUBA

Cocculus Palmatus
Jateorhiza calumba

Common name: Kalumb.

A bitter tonic free from astringent qualities and of great importance in the treatment of stomach conditions, especially where there is lack of appetite. It is indicated in debilitated conditions where the digestion is at fault. Combines well with Alfalfa seed for tea or an infusion.

Best taken as an infusion. One teaspoon of Caluba to a cup of boiling water, steep 30 minutes, and cool. Dose: 1 teaspoon in water before meals.

Dose of tincture: 20 to 40 drops in water, best before meals.

CASCARA SAGRADA

Rhamnus purshianus

Common name: California Buckthorn.

Called a childhood remedy, it is a very bitter tonic; a mild, slow, stimulating hepatic. Its influence is chiefly upon the stomach, liver, gall ducts, and, in a lesser degree, on the bowels. Its value is in chronic constipation, torpor of the stomach and liver, and chronic dyspepsia. It influences peristaltic action. Best given morning and evening.

A desirable means for the use or Cascara is by making:

Fluid Extract of Cascara Sagrada (*Rhamnus purshianus*)	1 ounce
Tincture of Butternut (*Juglans cinerea*)	¼ ounce
Simple Syrup (*Sugar and water*)	8 ounces

Dose: One tablespoon at bedtime and in the morning, if necessary.

Dose of tincture: 40 to 60 drops with water morning and evening according to need.

CHESTNUT, SWEET

Castanea vesca

Considered a specific in whooping cough, it is of great value in continued distressing coughs and in frequent hiccoughs.

It is best used as an infusion. One ounce to a pint of hot water steeped for one-half hour. One tablespoon or less for children, 2 tablespoons for adults, as frequently as necessary.

Dose of fluid extracts: 10 drops as indicated by condition.

The *Natura* physician sometimes combines *Lobelia* (Indian tobacco) and Blue Cohosh (Caulophyllum), as indicated by conditions.

CLIVERS

Galium aparine

Common names: Goosegrass, Cleaverwort, Bed Straw, Catchweed, Cleavers.

The agent for the treatment of inflammatory diseases of the kidneys, bladder, and urinary passages.

Galium is especially indicated in the latter stages of scarlet fever when there is a tendency to kidney irritation. In scalding urine it is *the* remedy.

Most effective when given as an infusion. It is made by steeping an ounce of cleavers in a pint of boiling water for several hours. Dose: 2 to 4 tablespoons, 4 times a day.

Dose of tincture: 20 to 40 drops in water 3 or 4 times a day, or as indicated by conditions.

DOGWOOD, AMERICAN

Cornus Florida

Common names: Box Wood, Flowering Cornel, Green Ozier.

Dogwood is a splendid substitute for quinine, its active principle being cornine. It has long been prized as a remedy in ague and similar ailments. It is effective as an infusion. It is made by steeping 1 tablespoon in a pint of boiling water for one-half hour, strain. Dose: one-half cup every 2 or 3 hours, or as indicated.

Tincture: 20 to 40 drops in water.

Cornus combines well with Peruvian Bark (Cinchona). In making an infusion, 1 tablespoon of Dogwood and 1 teaspoon of Peruvian Bark steeped in a pint of hot water for one-half hour, take 1 teaspoon in water every 2 or 3 hours, or more frequently if necessary.

ELDER, AMERICAN

Sambucus Canadensis

Common names: American Elder, Sweet Elder.

An anemia remedy. While American Elder has long been used as a family remedy and is of value in skin and febrile diseases, it is best known, and, most used, by making a cordial out of the berries and combining them with blackberries. These berries, as indicated by their color, are rich in organic iron and, therefore, of much benefit in anemia. Two ounces of the juice of the Elderberry and Blackberry combined, three or more times a day is of exceptional value in anemia.

It may be made into an infusion by steeping a teaspoon of the bark and root in a cup of hot water for one-half hour, 2 or more cups a day.

Dosage of the tincture: 20 to 40 drops in water 3 or 4 times a day.

An ointment made from the bark is of great value in the treatment of cuts, bruises, and various other sores. The salve is made by slowly heating a pound of finely cut elder bark in 2 pounds of lard and one-half pound of mutton suet, strain it. When cool, it is ready for use and may be kept for a long time. Other remedies for the same purpose may be combined with the bark.

GENTIAN, YELLOW

Gentiana Lutea

The ague remedy, Yellow Gentian is a bitter tonic and enters into a great many formulas in the treatment of the liver and various forms of dyspepsia.

Yellow Gentian is specifically an ague medicine and is frequently substituted for Quinine and will be effective when many other agents fail.

In cases where there are frequent chills, treatment should begin several hours before chills are again due.

In home use it is made into a syrup. One ounce each of gentain, ginger, and wahoo and 2 ounces of goldenseal, boneset, American Elder, and Coriander seeds for taste, and a small amount of orange peel for vitamin C are made into a syrup by steeping in a quart of boiling water for an hour, straining and mixing with a quart of simple syrup. Dosage: One teaspoon to a tablespoon every few hours according to age and condition.

Singly, it may be made into a semi-infusion, 2 ounces of the tops and roots to a pint of boiling water; steep for one-half hour. When cold, strain, and to this add one-half pint or more of good brandy. Dosage: From 1 to 2 teaspoons according to age and symptoms. Dose of the tincture: 5 to 10 drops in water before meals.

GUARANA

Pallinia Sorbilis

The Physio-Medical and *Natura* Physician's headache remedy. It is made into a fluid extract, a tincture, and an active principle, *Guaranine*. Although usually prescribed in either the fluid extract or tincture, it is not desirable as an infusion.

It can be depended on to give speedy relief in headache caused by mentally over-working, or as the result of exhaustive diseases where there is a tendency to faintness.

Dose of the fluid extract, 10 drops in water every half-hour for 3 doses. Dose of the tincture: 15 to 20 drops taken in the same way.

It is indicated in neuralgia caused by depression of the nervous system, taken in the same dosage and frequency. *Sorbilis* is *counterindicated in heart conditions.*

HOPS

Humulus Lupulus

Humulus is used for many purposes in medicine, but the two principal uses for it are as a hypnotic or in poultices.

In action, hops is a tonic, hypnotic, febrifuge, anthelmintic and may be prescribed for any of these purposes. It is essentially a family remedy.

It is best taken as an infusion by steeping a tablespoon or more of flowers in a cup of boiling water for one-half hour. Dosage: 1 tablespoon at a time, more at night as a hypnotic.

Dose of tincture: 5 to 20 drops in hot water.

For local application, hops is made into a hot fomentation and applied to the face to relieve facial and earache. As a poultice, it is applied to ease the pain in abscesses and bring them to a "head."

IGNATA AMARA

Strychnos Ignatii

Common name: Ignatius Beans.

A composite agent, it is a substitute for Strychnine. It is peculiarly a women's remedy and valuable if properly prescribed. Combines well with Pulsatilla given alternately. *Doses should be small.*

It is indicated when menses are dark or black, profuse or scanty, early rather than on time, melancholia, brooding over sorrows, hysteria, laughing or crying without real cause, neurotic, although mentally balanced, and sufferer is erratic and inconstant.

Dose: one-half to 2 drops as required. *To be taken only in emergencies or under the supervision of a physician.*

As associate agent with *Pulsatilla,* 1 to 2 drops, *taken separately.*

LINDEN FLOWERS

Tilia Europoea

Common name: Lime Tree, Common Lime.

Linden tea has long been used as a home remedy to promote perspiration in fevers and for relieving coughs and hoarseness during colds.

Infusion, or tea, is made by adding a teaspoon of the flowers and leaves to a cup of boiling water and steep for one-half hour. After cooling, a tablespoon in water as often as required. For inducing perspiration the infusion is taken in hot water.

Dose of tincture: 20 to 50 drops according to age and condition.

MANDRAKE, AMERICAN
Podophyllum peltatum

Common name: May Apple, Wild Lemon, Raccoon Berry.

May Apple is a cathartic, alterative, and anthelmintic. It is an active ingredient in many of the formulas for constipation. It is important because its action does not result in costiveness as do many other agents for this purpose.

In family usage, it is made into an infusion, a teaspoon of the root cut or powdered to a pint of boiling water, steep one-half hour. Dosage: 1 teaspoon as required.

Tincture: 2 to 5 drops in water. Dosage should *be carefully graded to requirements.*

MARSH MALLOW
Althaea officinalis

Chiefly a woman's remedy, although Marsh Mallow is much used in coughs due to colds and hoarseness too.

It is of real value as a tea in colitis. As a decoction used for vaginal douches, it is cleansing and soothing.

For infusion, a teaspoon of the powdered root is added to one-half pint of boiling water, steep for one-half hour, take 2 tablespoons every few hours. As a decoction for vaginal douches, an ounce is steeped in a quart of boiling water for an hour, strained, and used while slightly warm.

Dose of tincture: 20 to 40 drops.

PEACH TREE
Prunus Persica
Amygdalus Persica

The remedy for morning sickness in pregnancy.

The leaves of the peach tree are used in making the infusion, although the bark may also be used.

Amygalus is a sedative, bitters, aromatic, and a laxative when taken in large amounts.

The infusion is most generally used as a bitters to increase stomach functioning, and in jaundice and other liver affections, as well as an ingredient in whooping cough medication. It has proven generally effective in morning sickness of pregnancy and is certain to be free from harmful results. The dosage must be limited to the degree of normal bowel evacuation.

A teaspoon of the herb is steeped in a cup of boiling water for one-half hour and strained. Two or 3 cups a day may be taken as long as necessary.

Dose of tincture, 2 to 15 drops in water according to severity of the nausea. First dose on arising, other doses one-half hour before meals if necessary. The first cup of infusion also is taken before first meal of the day.

PERUVIAN BARK

Cinchona Succirubra

Common names: Foso Bark, Jesuits' Bark, Red Bark, Crown Bark, Cinchona.

One of the most important agents in malaria and in chills in colds and fevers. *It is not to be prescribed in pregnancies because of its possible oxytoxic effects.*

Cinchona is also a valuable agent in debilitating febrile conditions and as a tonic and stomachic. It should be taken in small doses except in emergencies where immediate reactions are desired.

An infusion may be made by steeping a teaspoon of the cut or powdered bark in 4 ounces of boiling water for one-half hour. Strain and take a teaspoon in water every 3 hours, or more frequently according to conditions and desired effect. As a family medicine, it took the place of Quinine.

Dose of the tincture, from 5 to 30 drops.

PINK ROOT

Spigelia Marilandica

Common names: Carolina Pink, Wormgrass.

The family worm medicine, one of the best and most non-poisonous domestic agents used as a vermifuge.

It is best given in an infusion by adding an ounce of the cut or powdered root in a pint of hot water and steeped for one-half hour. This is to be taken an ounce every hour, to be followed by a cathartic. Frequently, the housewife adds sufficient Senna in making the infusion for free bowel evacuation. Repeat: *Excessive doses or too strong cathartics are to be avoided.*

Instead of the infusion, 10 to 20 grains of the powder may be taken in hot water. Dosage depends on age.

QUEEN-OF-THE-MEADOW ROOT

Eupatorium Purpureum

Common names: Gravel Root, Joe-Pie-Weed, Trumpet Weed, Purple Boneset.

Eupatorium is a relaxing nervine, capable of soothing and increasing the action of the kidneys. It is of much value in irritable conditions of the bladder and in kidney conditions accompanied by aching in the small of the back. In irritated conditions of the female organs, it is most useful.

An infusion is made by steeping an ounce of cut root in a pint of hot water for one-half hour. Dosage: 1 ounce every 3 hours or as indicated.

Dose of tincture: 8 to 15 drops.

RED CLOVER

Trifolium Pratense

Trifolium is a contrivaral agent. In domestic use the blossoms have been gathered, dried, and used for tea in place of coffee or tea. Mothers have relied on it when their children were suffering with whooping cough or in general nervousness. The *Natura* physician prescribes it for this purpose in combination with other agents.

From times past it was considered a valuable agent in the treatment of scrofula and, therefore, as an associate agent with other agents in cancer, although never so recognized by the orthodox medical profession.

Extracts of red clover blossoms have been long and successfully used in the form of a salve for the removal of external cancer and the treatment of indolent ulcers, promoting granulation.

As an internal agent it is best given in infusion. One teaspoon of the blossom in a cup of boiling water, steeped for one-half hour, 3 to 4 times a day. Children get less of the amount in water as frequently as required.

Dose of the tincture: 5 to 30 drops in water according to age and purpose.

RED RASPBERRY

Rubus Strigosus

Common name: Wild Red Raspberry.

The root is used in the same manner as Blackberry and Dewberry Root. Combines well with them in making an infusion or syrup.

RUE

Rute graveolens

Common names: German Rue, Garden Rue, Herb-of-Grace, Countryman's Treacle (the last two names not in general usage).

This herb was used in domestic practice for centuries and even today is cultivated in many gardens. The entire plant, except the roots, is dried to be ready to make into an infusion in time of need.

It is a bitters and stimulant, mostly used for colic and gas pains, perfectly safe for home use. It has been—and is—still much used for cramps of menstruation in hot infusion and for general nervouseness and convulsions.

The infusion is made by steeping a teaspoon of the cut herb in a cup of boiling water for one-half hour and strain. For any form of cramps, one-third is added to a cup of hot water and taken every few hours until relieved. In other conditions it may be taken in cold water.

Dosage of tincture: 5 to 15 drops in hot or cold water depending on condition.

The infusion or tincture combines well with other agents indicated in similar condition.

ST. JOHN'S WORT, COMMON

Hypericum perforatum

Common name: John's Wort.

Hypericum is a soothing agent and was once found in almost every country household and used for general dyspepsia and other digestive disturbances. It was usually picked and placed into quart bottles, filled with good whisky, its virtues allowed to be extracted, then taken in 1 ounce portions before meals.

An infusion was frequently made for women and children by steeping 1 teaspoon of the powdered tops and flowers—or the green herb when in flower—to a cup of boiling water, steep for one-half hour, and take 2 tablespoons at a time.

Dosage of tincture: 8 to 15 drops in water before meals.

SARSAPARILLA, AMERICAN AND MEXICAN

Aralia Nudicaulis

Common names: Small Spikenard, Spignet.

Sarsaparilla has long been used in domestic practice with other agents used for the same purpose, i.e., loss or weakening of manhood. Its action alone is very feeble.

Within recent years Mexican Sarsaparilla root, or the tincture made from it, has been much publicized, and an untold number have been persuaded by great promises to pay rather large sums for it. Mexican Sarsaparilla has somewhat greater value than the American, but like the American it is of not much value unless combined with numerous agents for the same purpose.

Infusion is made with 2 ounces of the cut root to a pint of boiling water, steep an hour, and strain. Dose: 2 to 3 tablespoons, 3 or 4 times a day.

Dose of tincture: 20 to 40 drops, 4 times a day.

SHEEP'S SORREL

Rumex acetosella

Common names: Sourgrass, Red Sorrel, Field Sorrel.

The chief value of Sheep Sorrel is as an anti-scorbutic.

Its value is due to its richness in potassium. Potassium is of great improtance in the treatment of many serious blood infections including syphilis and cancer, and *now* to neutralize the effects of "fall-out." For this purpose it should be made into a salad in combination with raw cabbage, lettuce, tomatoes, spinach, and lightly boiled snap beans, all rich in potassium.

The infusion is made by steeping a teaspoon of the dried herb, or one-half teaspoon of the green herb, in a cup of boiling water for one-half hour, 2 or more cups a day.

The dosage of the tincture: 20 to 50 drops, 3 or 4 times a day.

SHEPHERD'S PURSE

Capsella bursa-pastoris

A stimulant, diuretic, and anti-scorbic, Shepherd's Purse is of much value in congested conditions of the kidneys and bladder, and in catarrh of the urinary tract indicated by much mucous in the urine.

Infusion is made by steeping a teaspoon of the herb in a cup of boiling water for one-half hour; 1 or 2 cups a day as required.

Dose of tincture: 20 to 40 drops, 2 to 3 times a day.

SKUNK-CABBAGE

Symplocarpus foetidus

Common names: Skunkweed, Polecatweed, Meadow Cabbage, Swamp Cabbage.

A well-known and long-used agent as a stimulant, expectorant, and antispasmodic, slightly narcotic. It is of much value in the spasms of asthma, whooping cough, nasal catarrh, and bronchial irritations. Only the root is used. For infusion, this is cut into small pieces, a teaspoon steeped in a cup of boiling water for one-half hour. When cold, a tablespoon at a time, as required.

Dosage of the tincture: 3 to 15 drops.

SLIPPERY ELM BARK

Ulnus fulva

Slippery Elm is probably best known by its long use in making poultices for various conditions. It is improved, if a small amount of glycerine is added.

Slippery Elm is likewise used in enemas, soothing to the lower bowels when inflammation is present, and for douches, reducing or eliminating vaginal inflammation. For either purpose an infusion is made by steeping 1 ounce of the cut bark in a quart of boiling water for an hour, strain it, and it is ready for use.

Slippery Elm possesses pronounced mucilaginous properties, making it a valuable agent in irritable or inflamed conditions of the mucous membranes, such as may be present in inflammations of the stomach, bowels, and kidneys. For this purpose 2 or more ounces of the bark should be steeped in a quart of boiling water for an hour or longer; strained, and used freely. The bark may be soaked for a much longer time, making it stronger and then mixed with honey or simple syrup. A teaspoon taken every half hour to soothe the membranes.

THYME, COMMON

Thymus vulgaris

Common name: Garden Thyme.

A domestic remedy for throat and bronchial irritation, and in spasms of whooping cough. It is useful in flatulence and colic, and effective in inducing free perspiration in the beginning of colds and in ordinary fever.

Infusion is made by adding a teaspoon of the herb in a cup of boiling water for one-half hour. Two or more cups a day, as indicated.

Dose of tincture: 20 to 50 drops in hot water.

TURTLE-HEAD

Chelone Glabra

Common names: Salt Rheum Seed, Belamony, Turtle-Bloom, Shell-flower.

The itching remedy. Internally, it is a tonic and has splendid affect on the liver, and a beneficial effect during convalescence.

Its most important use is as a salve to relieve the itching of chickenpox and measles. It is made by adding the leaves, 2 or more ounces to one-half pound of lard, and boiling slowly for 30 minutes. Strain, cool, and it is ready for use. It is equally allaying in itching piles.

For internal use, an infusion is made by steeping a teaspoon of the herb in a cup of boiling water for one-half hour, 1 or more cups a day.

Dosage of tincture: 20 to 50 drops.

VIRGINIA SNAKEROOT

Aristolochia serpentaria

Common names: Red River Snakeroot, Texas Snakeroot, Sangrel, Sangreeroot.

The stomach bitters, a man's remedy. This agent has been used as a stomach bitters since time unrecorded. The fresh root is placed in a bottle, filled with good whiskey, and permitted to stand for a week, shaking occasionally. Dose: 1 ounce, or even more, before meals. This agent has already been considered. Due to its former general and present use, it deserves special consideration.

Dose of tincture: 1 to 20 drops in water. *To be used with caution.*

WHITE PINE

Pinus Strobus
Pinus Alba

Common names: Deal Pine, Soft Pine.

An excellent expectorant, to reduce the mucous secretions frequent in common colds and help in its elimination.

An infusion is made by steeping 1 teaspoon of the White Pine in a pint of boiling water for one-half hour. When cool, take 1 or 2 tablespoons as often as necessary to relieve the condition.

The infusion is made by steeping White Pine, or the combination following: 1 teaspoon in a pint of boiling water, steep for one-half hour. When cool, take 1 or 2 tablespoons as indicated by condition.

Dose of tincture, 2 to 10 drops in water.

White Pine is best combined with Wild Cherry (*Prunus Virginiana*), Sassafras, (*Laurus*), and Spikenard (*Aralia Racemosa*), 1 tablespoon each to the 1 teaspoon of Wihte Pine in a pint of boiling water for one-half hour, 1 teaspoon or more every hour or two to eliminate the condition.

White Pine substitutes for the creosote commonly used in cough remedies.

WILD CHERRY BARK

Prunus Serotina

Common names: Choke Cherry, Rum Cherry.

Long used as a valued ingredient in cough remedies. It is combined with neutralizing cordials and is indicated in indigestion caused by lack of tone in the stomach.

A favorite combination much used by men with digestive difficulties is to fill a quart bottle half full with the broken bark and cherries, and then add good whisky or brandy. Shake frequently. After a week, a tablespoon or more before meals.

Dose of the tincture: 10 to 15 drops with water.

In chronic coughs, a formula containing:

Tincture of Wild Cherry Bark (*Prunus Serotina*)	2 ounces
Tincture of Spikenard (*Aralia racemosa*)	1 ounce
Tincture of Lippia (*Lippia dulcis*)	½ ounce

Dosage: 10 to 20 drops as indicated. This formula may be added to a pint of simple syrup. Dosage: one teaspoon as necessary.

WINTERGREEN

Gaultheria procumbens

Common names: Checkerberry, Periwinkle, Spice Berry, Deerberry, Teaberry.

The oil of Wintergreen is one of the most useful and potent agents as an external application to relieve pain of almost every nature.

Gaultheria is frequently prescribed in the form of oil, or other media, in rheumatism and other conditions of like nature in dose of 6 to 8 drops. *It is best that the oil be taken only when prescribed by a physician.*

The plant may be cut or powdered and made into an infusion. A teaspoon of it in a cup of boiling water, steep one-half hour, strain, and take in tablespoonful doses throughout the day.

Dose of tincture: 5 to 15 drops.

WITCH HAZEL

Hamamelis virginiana

A universally used home remedy for many purposes. In internal medication it is useful in dystentery. Valuable as a wash for sore mouth, inflamed eyes, burns, bruises, skin irritations, and other forms of external inflammation. The distilled non-alcholic form is to be preferred.

An infusion may be made by steeping the bark or leaves, or a combination of them, in a cup of boiling water. When cold, divide into 3 portions; one portion morning, noon, or night.

Dose of the tincture: 5 to 20 drops, according to age and/or condition.

11.

THE NATURA TREATMENT OF DISEASE

The following selected simplified formulas or prescriptions are from the author's notebook; the final choice is based on the generally successful treatment of the diseases named.

This simplification is considered desirable because many, in fact in almost all of the agents (remedies) described, are in the physician's Armamentarium where detailed descriptions and the most essential properties are given in the treatment of various diseases indicated.

ACIDOSIS
General Systemic Acid Condition

Tincture of Motherwort (*Leonurus cardiaca*)	10 to 20 drops
Tincture of Water Cress (*Nasturtium Officinale*)	10 to 20 drops
Tincture of Sweet Flag (*Acorus Calamus*)	10 to 20 drops
Tincture of Goldenseal (*Hydrastis canadensis*)	6 to 10 drops

In water before meals, Charcoal tablets between meals.

In domestic practice it has been and continues to be, the practice to steep a teaspoon of Motherwort, Water Cress, Sweet Flag and three-quarters of a teaspoon of Goldenseal (all dried) in a pint of water for 30 minutes. Strain, bottle, and add sufficient brandy to prevent fermentation. Dose: 1 tablespoon before meals. Charcoal tablets between meals.

AGUE
Intermittent Fever—Chills and Fever

Tincture of Goldenseal (*Hydrastis canadensis*)	6 to 12 drops
Tincture of Gentian (*Gentiana lutes*)	15 to 29 drops
Tincture of Fringe Tree (*Chiolanthus virginica*)	3 to 7 drops
Tincture of Cayenne Pepper (*Capsicum frutescens*)	1 to 3 drops

In water every 1 or 2 hours according to severity of symptoms. The diet is important. Plenty of vegetables, both raw and boiled, (rich in organic iron) should be part of every meal.

Tincture of Goldenseal (*Hydrastis canadensis*)	8 to 12 drops
Tincture of Squaw Vine (*Mitchella repens*)	6 to 15 drops
Tincture of Peruvian Bark (*Cinchona succiruba*)	1 to 2 drops

In water before meals. Organic iron should be prescribed in conjunction with this formula.

ANEMIA

General Physical Weakness Tonic

Tincture of Bayberry (*Myrica cerifera*)	5 to 10 drops
Tincture of Goldenseal (*Hydrastis canadensis*)	7 to 9 drops
Tincture of Pasque Flower (*Anenome pulsatilla*)	1 to 2 drops
Tincture of Oat Beards (*Avena sativa*)	12 to 20 drops

In water before meals.

In addition, organic iron and raw and boiled vegetables rich in iron—at least twice a day.

In anemia the diet is generally, if not always, at fault—too low in iron (and other organic minerals) and vital elements. Sanitation is poor; this *must* have careful attention, if treatment is to be successful.

ANGINA PECTORIS

Chest Spasms—Breast Pang

Tincture of Cayenne Pepper (*Capsicum frutescens*)	2 to 4 drops
Tincture of Indian Tobacco (*Lobelia inflata*)	10 to 15 drops

In water every 30 to 45 minutes according to symptoms.

Cayenne Pepper is best given in tablet form at the same time as Indian Tobacco is given in water. Repeat every 30 minutes, if necessary, to stop spasms.

APPENDICITIS, CHRONIC

Tincture of Lady's Slipper (*Cypripedium pubescens*)	8 to 15 drops
Tincture of Indian Tobacco (*Lobelia inflata*)	10 to 20 drops

In water every 30 minutes during attacks of pain. Follow with treatment for intestinal congestion.

ASTHMA

Phthisic Spasmodic Breathing

During attacks:

Tincture of Indian Tobacco (*Lobelia inflata*)	10 to 20 drops
Tincture of Black Haw (*Viburnum opulus*)	5 to 10 drops

In water every 3 or 4 hours for the duration of the attacks, followed by general treatment, which should include small doses of Cayenne Pepper.

ATAXIA

Tabes Dolsalis

For proper treatment, cause must be found. These are varied from blood diseases to accidents.

ACUTE ATTACKS

Tincture of Indian Tobacco (*Lobelia inflata*)	20 to 30 drops
Tincture of Cayenne Pepper (*Capsicum frutescens*)	2 to 4 drops

Take every half hour as necessary. Cayenne Pepper is best given in tablet form, the Indian Tobacco with water.

GENERAL TREATMENT

Tincture of Great Mullein (*Verbascum thapsus*)	10 drops

This has proven most successful as a general treatment. Dose: 10 drops in water, three times a day.

BED WETTING

Enuresis

Bed wetting may be either a habit or due to some weakness, usually of a nervous nature, and should be treated accordingly.

A general formula of much value:

Tincture of Agrimony (*Agrimonia eupatoria*)	3 to 8 drops
Tincture of Corn Silk (*Stigmata maydis*)	5 to 15 drops
Tincture of Lady's Slipper (*Cypripedium pubescens*)	10 to 20 drops
Tincture of Shepherd's Purse (*Capsella bursa-pastoris*)	20 to 30 drops

Dose: divide into two portions, one at noon and the other at bed-time. For adults, the full amount, two or three times a day; the last at retiring.

This may be made into an infusion by steeping equal parts in a quart of boiling water for an hour, strain, add 2 pounds of brown sugar and an ounce of glycerine. Dose: one teaspoon before meals and on retiring.

Between meals, 5 drops of Great mullein oil in water for children; 10 drops for adults. No liquids before retiring.

BRIGHT'S DISEASE

Albuminuria

Except in emergencies, there should be a careful examination and search for the cause of the condition and treatment arranged accordingly. All stimulating liquids are to be avoided. Elimination from skin, kidneys, and bowels encouraged. General treatment to be changed according to condition:

A favorite formula long prescribed by physio-medical and natura physicians with generally good results consists of:

Fluid extract of Seven Barks (*Hydrangea arborescens*)	1 ounce
Fluid extract of Couch-Grass (*Triticum repens*)	½ ounce
Fluid extract of Hollyhock (*Althaea rosea*)	½ ounce
Mucilage of Gum Arabic	1½ ounces
Glycerine	½ ounce

Dose: 1 teaspoon a day for 3 to 5 days. Following with agents indicated for the condition. Repeat. Surgery may be necessary in emergency conditions.

BRONCHITIS

Bronchial Catarrh

Tincture of Indian Tobacco (*Lolbeia inflata*)	3 to 5 drops
Tincture of Milkweed (*Asclepias cornuti*)	5 to 10 drops
Tincture of Queen's Root (*Stillingia sylvatica*)	7 to 10 drops

Dose: 3 or more times a day in water according to condition. Dosage may be increased.

If a putrid condition develops (easily recognized by the odor of the sputum), 2 grains of tincture of myrrh should be added to the formula.

Chronic Bronchitis

For the cough of chronic bronchitis where it is loose and expectoration free:

Tincture of Spikenard (*Aralia racemosa*)	10 to 15 drops
Tincture of Black Haw (*Viburnum opulus*)	10 to 15 drops
Tincture of Hops (*Humulus lupulus*)	20 to 30 drops

Dose: 3 or 4 times a day.

An infusion may be made with the herbs: 2 ounces Spikenard, 1 ounce Black Haw, and 3 ounces Hops steeped in one pint of boiling water for one-half hour. Steep, strain, and add 3 ounces of honey.

Dose: One tablespoon frequently—as required.

CALCULI (URINARY)

Stone in Bladder and/or Kidneys

The diet must be light, nourishing, but no rich soups for best results.

Tincture of Scullcap (*Scutellaria Lateriflora*)	3 to 6 drops
Tincture of Pleurisy Root (*Asclepias tuberose*)	6 to 12 drops

Dose: in hot water every 3 or 4 hours if there is temperature.

Instead of the tincture, a very desirable and effective infusion is made of 1 ounce Scullcap and one-half ounce of Pleurisy Root steeped in a pint of boiling water, strained, and a little honey added.

Dose: 1 tablespoon in hot water every few hours. This is especially important if the skin is hot.

For itching, which is practically always present, and to prevent scratching: Use 2 ounces Indian Tobacco, 7 ounces of extract of Witch hazel, in a pint of hot water. If there should happen to be the formation of pus, one-half ounce of tincture of myrrh is added to this solution.

With care, practically no internal medication will be necessary except the teas frequently given. Elimination kept normal.

CANCER

Because of its controversial nature, cancer, like diabetes and high blood pressure, must be given different consideration than the various other diseases.

GAULTHERIA (PERIWINKLE)

Gaultheria has already been considered in a different manner as an agent in the treatment of various diseases. At the present moment it is separated from, or as a means of, general medication and receives special consideration as an agent in the treatment of various forms of cancer. Due to the fact that it is a controversial agent not generally acknowledged as possessing any virtue as such an agent, there is no pretension on our part that it will "cure" cancer despite the fact that we know it to have been successful in some cases.

The *Tucson Citizen,* April 11, 1960, reported results of experiments with this agent for the purpose.

"The scientists (making the experiments) said 'encouraging anti-cancer properties in man and animals' were exhibited by substances from the plant.

"The groups, headed by M. E. Hordes, Indiana University; Roy Hertz, National Cancer Institute; and Gordon H. Svoboda, Lilly Laboratories, presented their findings at the Association's annual meeting.

"The report stated the properties were found in a class of chemicals used in cancer clinics for the first time. One of these is a newly discovered alkaloid of periwinkle known as *Vincaleukoblastin,* commonly called VLB.

"Their reports said preliminary clinical trials involving about 30 patients showed that VLB sulfate produced:

Improvement in various acute leukemias, some resistance to other cancer drugs.

Suppression of the growth and activity of certain solid tumors on the placenta called carcinomas.

"The new class of experimental anti-cancer agents, the scientists said, was of unusual interest to scientists because anti-cancer chemicals of plant origin are rare in medicine. They said the discovery is likely to stimulate much wider investigation of the plant for anti-cancer activity."

Throughout the years, physicians of all schools have guardedly claimed curing cancer by various means of herbal medication.

The Natura physician usually prescribes an infusion of the plant made by steeping a teaspoonful of the cut or granulated plant in a cup of boiling water for one-half hour; strain. One tablespoon frequently during the day.

Dosage of the tincture is 5 to 10 drops in cold water 4 times a day.

Red Clover (*Trifolium pratense*) 1 teaspoon of the flowers steeped in a cup of boiling water for one-half hour; strain. One cup during the day.

Dosage of tincture 20 to 40 drops.

Comfrey (Symphytum officinale), 1 ounce of the powdered roots in one cup of boiling water; steep for one-half hour and strain. Divide into 4 parts; 1 part, 4 times a day.

Dosage of tincture 10 to 40 drops in water.

Coneflower (*Echinacea*) 1 ounce of the cut root steeped in 1 cup of boiling water for one-half hour, and strain. Divide into 3 portions, 1 part, 3 times a day.

Dosage of tincture 10 to 30 drops.

The infusions have long been used, but the procedure is tedious, though necessary, where tinctures are not procurable. Tinctures are standardized and more certain and should be substituted for the infusions where possible:

Tincture of Periwinkle	5 to 10 drops
Tincture of Coneflower (*Echinacea angustiflora*)	15 to 30 drops
Tincture of Comfrey (*Symphytum officinale*)	10 to 40 drops
Tincture of Red Clover (*Trifolium pratense*)	20 to 40 drops

In water 4 times a day.

Diet must be carefully selected. No denatured sugars or starches. Carefully selected protein. Plenty of fresh vegetables, rich in potassium. All foods heavy with congesting material must be avoided. The liver must be kept active by proper medication. Elimination free.

CATARRH
Chronic (General)

Tincture of Blazing Star	8 to 12 drops
Tincture of Scullcap	2 to 4 drops
Tincture of Blue Cohosh	5 to 10 drops
Tincture of Golden Seal	8 to 10 drops

Three or more times a day.

Catarrh is not a disease in itself. While treating it, the cause should be found and eliminated, and food elements supplied which will remove the cause.

CATARRH OF THE BLADDER
Cystitis—Vesicular Catarrh

Tincture of Bearberry	5 to 20 drops
Tincture of Peach Tree Leaves	5 to 10 drops

Dose: Take in water three or more times a day according to symptoms.

In chronic conditions, 5 drops of tincture of *barosma* (buchu) should be added.

In acute Cystitis this formula is generally effective:

Tincture of Marsh Mallow	10 to 15 drops
Tincture of Couch-Grass	10 to 20 drops
Tincture of Shepherd's Purse	10 to 20 drops

Dose: divide into 3 portions. One between each meal and at bedtime. Dosage may be increased according to condition.

All alcohol must be forbidden as are also highly seasoned foods.

An infusion of much value may be made of the marsh mallow, couch grass and shepherd's purse—one-half ounce each steeped in 1 quart of boiling water for 30 minutes or more; strain; use one-half cupful every 3 hours.

A favorite formula of many physicians is composed of:

Tincture of Corn Silk	10 to 15 drops
Tincture of Colic Root	8 to 12 drops

Dose: Three or 4 times a day or more frequently as required.

If pus shows in the urine, 1 drop of Tincture of *myrrh* should be added to each dose.

CHICKEN POX

Varicella

This childhood disease is a simple one if correctly treated, otherwise, there may be serious complications.

Bed at first symptoms. Even temperature. Elimination by skin and bowels. Avoid all draft and chills. Temperature treated with teas: Pennyroyal, Catnip, Mint and/or fruit juices.

If the stomach is upset, this should have immediate attention lest there be an increase of temperature.

Tincture of Marsh Mallow (*Althea officinale*)	10 drops
Tincture of Peach Tree Leaves (*Prunus Persica*)	5 to 10 drops
Tincture of Pleurisy Root (*Asclepias tuberose*)	5 to 10 drops

Three or 4 times a day according to condition.

CHLOROSIS—ANEMIA OF PUBERTY

Green Sickness

With proper diet this ailment, formerly so prevalent with modern endocrine (glandular) treatment, should be readily prevented from becoming serious.

Medication must have in view building up the vital and resistant forces of the body. General medication will help prevent the development of the condition.

Infusions are more effective than the tinctures:

Scullcap (*Scutellaria Lateriflora*)	1 ounce
Blue Cohosh (*Caulophyllum thalictroides*)	1 ounce
Goldenseal (*Hydrastis canadensis*)	½ ounce
Coriander Seed (*Coriandrum sativum*)	½ ounce
Orange Peel	½ ounce

Mix herbs, seed, and peel, and steep in 1 quart of boiling water, strain and add 1 pound of sugar and 2 ounces of glycerine.

A teaspoon or more after each meal and on retiring.

CHOLERA INFANTUM

Summer Complaint in Children

Cholera infantum is to be considered an emergency illness requiring the immediate attention of a physician because of its rapid development. Refer to physician's Armamentarium.

Patient must have absolute quietness. No annoyance of any kind. At first sign of temperature, cool drinks. Food requires utmost care. Malted milk is to be preferred above all other foods. Ceylon (generally known as India tea), brewed 5 minutes and given when cool is of benefit because of the tannin content.

Tincture of Raspberry Leaves (*Rubus Idaeus*)	20 to 40 drops
Tincture of Marsh Mallow (*Althea officinale*)	15 to 40 drops
Tincture of Comfrey (*Symphytum officinale*)	15 to 30 drops

In water as frequently as necessary, indicated by condition. If pus or blood appears in stool, add 4 to 6 drops of tincture of Myrrh.

This infusion may be given instead:

Raspberry Leaves (*Rubus Idaeus*)	1 ounce
Marsh Mallow (*Althea officinale*)	1 ounce
Comfrey (*Symphytum officinale*)	1 ounce

Steep in one pint of boiling water for one-half hour and strain. Dose: one teaspoon every hour in warm water. May be added to Catnip tea instead of warm water.

During convalescence Wild Cherry syrup is of benefit. Gradual return to regular diet.

In earlier times, even now in rural districts, family medication placed great dependence on Blackberry root and Red Raspberry leaves infusion.

COLIC

Children

Colic—stomach pains—in children, are multitudinous. Unless caused by some more serious illness they are simple in their treatment, and the remedies for their treatment were formerly known to practically every mother. The remedies were in the form of gathered dried herbs, readily at hand. These were: chamomile (in itself generally depended on for many conditions), Pennyroyal, Spearmint, Catniu, Peppermint, Ginger, Fennel.

As a rule, they were used singly, made into a tea or infusion, but would readily combine.

Chamomile—teaspoon steeped in a cup of boiling water for one-half hour. Strain, cool. One teaspoon every hour.

Pennyroyal—teaspoon steeped in cup of boiling water for one-half hour. Cool. One teaspoon, or more every hour or oftener.

Spearmint—One Teaspoon steeped in a cup of boiling water for one-half hour. Steep, cool. One teaspoon every 2 hours.

Peppermint—One teaspoon steeped in boiling water for one-half hour. Strain. One teaspoon every hour.

Ginger—One teaspoon steeped in boiling water for one-half hour. Strain. One teaspon in water every hour. Tincture may be used instead of infusion: 10 to 30 drops in water.

Fennel—One-half teaspoon of seed in a cup of boiling water for 1 hour. Steep. One teaspoon every hour.

Frequency of giving any one of these teas or infusions depends on severity of condition. Teas made one-half strength may be given in much larger amounts.

In modern practice the natura physician prescribes any *one* of these herbals in tincture form, selecting the agent best indicated:

Tincture of Ginger (*Zingiber officinale*)	5 to 10 drops
Tincture of Chamomile (*Anthemis nobilis*)	15 to 40 drops
Tincture of Pennyroyal (*Mentha pulegium*)	1 to 5 drops
Tincture of Spearmint (*Mentha viridis*)	5 to 15 drops
Tincture of Catnip (*Nepeta cataria*)	10 to 20 drops
Tincture of Fennel (*Foeniculum vulgare*)	10 to 20 drops

Dosage and frequency according to age and severity of attack, always in warm water.

CONSTIPATION

General Treatment

Natura materia medica is replete with remedies for this almost universal condition (habit), and medication should be chosen according to cause and associated conditions.

A simple treatment where persistaltic action is weak is:

Cascara Sagrada: 10 or more drops in water, night and morning. This should not be continued long because the system adjusts to it and there is lack of activity in the agent.

An infusion made into a syrup containing:

Butternut Bark (*Juglans cinerea*)	½ pound
Wahoo (*Euonymus atropurpureus*)	2 ounces
Goldenseal (*Hydrastis canadensis*)	2 ounces
Peppermint (*Mentha piperita*)	1 ounce

Steep in boiling water for 1 hour. Strain. Add 1 pound sugar and 2 ounces glycerine. Dose: one teaspoon or more as necessary, night and morning. Tinctures may be substituted in general practice:

Tincture of Butternut Bark (*Juglans cinerea*)	8 drops
Tincture of Wahoo (*Euonymus atropurpureus*)	5 drops
Tincture of Goldenseal (*Hydrastis canadensis*)	7 drops

Dosage: more or less according to age and condition, night and morning.

CORYZA

Coryza, with temperature, is frequently diagnosed as la grippe or influenza. The treatment is practically the same, with variations, according to symptoms:

Tincture of Carolina Jasmine (*Gelsemium nitidum*)	2 to 3 drops
Tincture of Boneset (*Eupatorium perfoliatum*)	10 to 20 drops
Tincture of Pleurisy Root (*Asclepias tuberose*)	12 to 20 drops
Tincture of Peruvian Bark (*Cinchona succirubra*)	1 to 10 drops

In water every 2 or 3 hours according to condition.

CROUP

Pseudo-Membranous or Inflammatory

Croup must always be considered an emergency condition and means taken to relieve the condition. Consult Physician's Armamentarium.

The *Natura* physician's first choice for immediate action still remains Thomson's third preparation in water every 15 minutes until vomiting and relaxation occur. After vomiting a lesser dosage every one-half hour. Where suffocation appears imminent, increase dosage.

General medication:

Tincture of Pleurisy Root (*Asclepias tuberose*)	30 to 60 drops
Tincture of Ginger (*Zingiber officinale*)	15 to 50 drops
Tincture of Indian Tobacco (*Lobelia inflata*)	2 to 4 drops

Dosage and frequency according to condition. Always in hot water.

For the cough:

Tincture of Wild Cherry Bark (*Prunus Serotina*)	10 to 20 drops
Tincture of Black Haw (*Viburnum opulus*)	8 to 10 drops

Dosage increased or reduced according to age and condition.
Treatment must be vigorous and constant.

DEMENTIA

Neurosis During Change of Life

In all too numerous instances, due to many causes present in modern life, various neurotic conditions develop during menopause. Recognizable symptoms appear and, if prompt attention is paid them, serious consequences may be avoided. Among the most important remedies are: Lady's Slipper, Pasque Flower, Passion Flower, and Motherwort.

Tincture of Pasque Flower (*Anenome pulsatilla*)	1 to 2 drops
Tincture of Lady's Slipper (*Cypripedium pubescens*)	5 to 10 drops
Tincture of Motherwort (*Leonurus cardiaca*)	10 to 20 drops
Tincture of Passion Flower (*Passiflora incarnata*)	10 to 20 drops

In water 3 or 4 times a day. More frequent if necessary.

DIABETES INSIPIDUS

Polyuria

The Physio-medical treatment generally consisted of:

Citric Acid	20 grains
Tartrate of Iron and Potassa	20 grains
Glycerine	1 ounce

Dissolve in 7 ounces of water. Dose: 1 teaspoon after each meal.

The natura general treatment may be in combination with the physio-medical formula:

Tincture of Corn Silk (*Stigmata Maydis*)	15 to 30 drops
Tincture of Scullcap (*Scutellaria Lateriflora*)	2 to 20 drops
Tincture of Wild Cherry Bark (*Prunus Serotina*)	20 to 40 drops
Tincture of Pipsissewa (*Chimaphila Umbellata*)	1 to 15 drops

In water 3 to 4 times a day.

DIABETES MELLITUS

Saccharine or Sugary Urine

In the treatment of diabetes, diet is of *utmost* importance *and must be consistently followed*. Condition of the stomach, liver, and elimination must be strictly attended to.

Physio-medical treatment:

Tartrate of Iron	1 ounce
Potassa	1 ounce
Citric Acid	1 ounce
Glycerine	1 ounce
Water	7 ounces

Dose: 1 teaspoon before meals.

Natura treatment:

Tincture of False Unicorn Root (*Chamaelirium luteum*)	2 ounces
Tincture of Coneflower (*Echinacea angustifolia*)	2 ounces

This combination is most effective, if it is combined with an infusion made with 4 ounces of Blueberry leaves steeped in a pint of boiling water for one-half hour and strained. Dosage: 1 to 2 tablespoons, 3 or 4 times a day.

Instead of the infusion, 2 ounces of the tincture of Blueberry may be added to the formula. Dosage: 20 to 30 drops, 3 or 4 times a day.

DIARRHOEA

If the liver is at fault:

Tincture of Goldenseal (*Hydrastis canadensis*)	7 to 10 drops

In water before meals.

Between meals and before retiring:

Tincture of Poplar (*Populus tremuloides*)	5 to 10 drops
Tincture of Rhubarb	3 to 5 drops
Tincture of Witch Hazel (*Hamemalis virginiana*)	10 to 20 drops

Dosage: according to condition.

If there is a decided odor, add 1 to 3 drops of tincture of myrrh.

If there is great nervous tension:

Tincture of Scullcap (*Scutellaria Lateriflora*)	8 to 15 drops
Tincture of Bayberry	8 to 15 drops

Every 3 hours. Dosage in all cases must be according to age and seriousness of condition. Diet must be light and neutral: rice, okra, and malted milk.

Chronic

Tincture of Poplar (*Populus tremuloides*)	8 to 15 drops
Tincture of Witch Hazel (*Hamemalis virginiana*)	8 to 15 drops
Tincture of Bayberry	8 to 13 drops

Every 3 or 4 hours. Dosage according to age and condition.

DIPHTHERIA

Malignant Sore Throat

An emergency infectious disease requiring immediate and careful attention. Consult physician's Armamentarium.

Any infection of the throat accompanied with temperature—though this is not always present in the beginning—should be suspected and receive prompt attention.

The most effective natura treatment is the Thomson course of treatment in association with other agents. Treatment must be vigorous:

Tincture of Goldenseal (*Hydrastis canadensis*)	8 to 15 drops
Tincture of Scullcap (*Scutellaria Lateriflora*)	10 to 15 drops

Dosage: according to age and condition every 2 to 3 hours. If the breath is putrid, 1 or 2 drops of tincture of myrrh.

Instead of the tincture, an infusion may be made:

Goldenseal (*Hydrastis canadensis*)	½ ounce
Scullcap (*Scutellaria Lateriflora*)	½ ounce

Steep in one pint of boiling water. Strain and add one-quarter teaspoon of tincture of myrrh. Dosage: 2 teaspoons every 2 hours, or as indicated by condition.

Gargle should be frequent and composed of borax and tincture of myrrh in water, or some other effective antiseptic agents.

An effective spray is made of:

Tincture of Goldenseal (*Hydrastis canadensis*)	½ ounce
Tincture of Myrrh (*Commiphora myrrha*)	10 drops

Every hour or more frequently.

The age-old domestic external application is still effective in the various throat affections: a woolen cloth about the throat. On an additional cloth the kerosene or turpentine lightly sprayed and placed over the first cloth. This should *not* be strong enough to blister.

Suspect any form of throat infection and treat promptly and effectively.

DROPSY

Anasarca Ascites

The natura physician does not consider dropsy an initial disease, but one caused by various other organic disorders which must have first or associate treatment. General treatment:

Tincture of Shepherd's Purse (*Capsella bursa-pastoris*)	10 to 18 drops
Tincture of Corn Silk (*Stigmata Maydis*)	8 to 15 drops

If there is associated constipation:

Tincture of Butternut (*Juglans cinerea*)	3 to 5 drops

According to requirement, every 2 to 3 hours.

Where possible, an infusion should be regularly given composed of:

Goldenseal Powdered Root (*Hydrastis canadensis*)	1 teaspoon
Peach Tree Leaves (*Prunus Persica*)	2 teaspoons

Steeped in 5 ounces of boiling water for 30 minutes. Strain. One tablespoon every 3 hours.

Associated treatment:

Tincture of Pipsissewa (*Chimaphila Umbellata*)	1 to 10 drops
Tincture of Poplar (*Populus tremuloides*)	1 to 10 drops
Tincture of Dwarf Elder (*Sambuccus Ebulus*)	5 to 10 drops
Tincture of Dandelion	10 to 20 drops

Dosage: in water 3 to 4 times a day, according to symptoms.

DYSENTERY

Diarrhoea

Any type of dysentery with which cramps are associated should receive prompt attention lest it turn into dangerous bloody flux. Rest, no irritating liquids, and simple food such as soups, malted milk, or milk brought to a near boil in which a beaten white of egg is mixed.

A simple and usually effective combination is:

Tincture of Bayberry (*Myrica cerifera*)	5 drops
Tincture of Poplar (*Populus tremuloides*)	5 drops
Tincture of Red Raspberry (*Rubus idaeus*)	5 drops
Tincture of Blackberry (*Rubus villosus*)	5 to 10 drops

Dosage: in water every 2 to 3 hours. An ounce of the roots and barks may be steeped for one-half hour and strained. A tablespoon of the infusion every 2 or 3 hours.

Note: Blackberry is often confused with Raspberry. Blackberry is a very low growing form. The roots are used in tinctures or infusion. It is of greater value in dysentery, especially in children, than the Raspberry.

In the more advanced stages of dysentery, 3 drops of tincture of Myrrh and/or tincture of cranesbill 5 to 10 drops should be added. In severe cases, use both.

If there is blood in the stool, 2 ounces of the infusion to which is added 4 drops of Tincture of Myrrh; 20 drops of Cranesbill and 1 ounce of witch Hazel should be added to a quart of slightly warm water and use as an enema every 4 hours, or as necessary, to help relieve the condition.

Extreme care should exercised in the treatment of these cases.

During Pregnancy

Unless the condition is severe, the first formula should be given to which is added 5 to 10 drops of Squaw Vine every 3 or 4 hours as condition demands.

DYSPEPSIA

Indigestion—General Catarrh

There are causes too numerous to mention that create this condition. In each instance, the cause should be found, treated and removed. Treatment is general:

Tincture of Hope (*Humulus Lubulus*)	5 to 10 drops
Tincture of Ginger (*Zingiber officinale*)	5 to 15 drops

In 3 ounces of water one-half hour after meals, or:

Tincture of Golenseal (*Hydrastis canadensis*)	5 to 10 drops
Tincture of Jersey Tea (*Ceanothus americanus*)	4 to 7 drops
Tincture of Fringe Tree (*Chiolanthus virginica*)	3 to 7 drops

In 3 ounces of water directly after meals or one-half hour before meals, or:

Tincture of Goldenseal (*Hydrastis canadensis*)	7 to 10 drops
Tincture of Yellow Gentian (*Gentiana lutea*)	10 to 15 drops
Tincture of Bitter Root (*Apocynum Androsaemifolium*)	5 to 8 drops
Tincture of St. John's Wort (*Hypericum perforatum*)	8 drops

In 3 ounces of water after meals.

An infusion may be made with 1 ounce Goldenseal, 3 ounces of Bitter Root and 2 ounces of St. John's Wort steeped in a pint of boiling water. Every one-half hour. Dose: one-half to 1 ounce of the infusion in 3 ounces of water after meals.

Tincture of Scullcap (*Scutellaria Laterifolia*)	5 to 15 drops
Tincture of Lady's Slipper (*Cypripedium pubescens*)	5 to 15 drops

DYSURIA

Difficult Urination

The causes are numerous, and must be found and treated with the agents herein noted and indicated for the purpose. In many instances the cause may be extremely serious and should receive prompt and careful attention. Consult physician's Armamentarium.

ECZEMA

Tetter-Sault Rheum and Other Skin Diseases

The causes of skin affection are many and frequently due to an extremely faulty diet and very poor elimination. The cause should be found, corrected, and proper agents prescribed and external manifestations properly treated.

A formula frequently effective for internal treatment:

Tincture of Bitter Sweet (*Solanum Dulcamara*)	5 to 10 drops
Tincture of Coneflower (*Echinacea angustifolia*)	10 to 15 drops
Tincture of Bittersweet	5 to 10 drops
Tincture of Burdock	5 to 15 drops
Tincture of Rhubarb	3 to 6 drops

In 3 ounces of water two or three times a day, in severe cases (less in milder cases) or:

Tincture of Goldenseal (*Hydrastis canadensis*)	7 to 10 drops
Tincture of Burdock	5 to 15 drops
Tincture of Queen's Root	3 to 9 drops
Tincture of Dandelion	10 to 15 drops

In 4 ounces of water two or three times a day.

As an external application in the treatment of eczema and similar skin diseases, an infusion made of Chamomile, 1 tablespoon of the herb to a cup of boiling water for 1 hour then drained and frequently applied, has been very successful. A salve may be made of it by boiling it in lard slowly for 15 minutes; after draining and cooling, it is ready to use. Tincture Marigold may be combined with it.

ENDOCARDITIS

Inflammation of the Heart's Lining Membrane

To be considered as a serious condition. Usually associated with, or following such conditions as Bright's disease, acute infectious scarlet fever, measles, child-bed fevers and poisonous irritants in the blood. Efforts must be to remove the cause and allay the inflammation.

Tincture of Virginia Snakeroot (*Aristolochia Serpentaria*)	5 drops

In water every 3 hours, or:

An infusion made of 1 tablespoon of cut or powdered roots steeped in 5 ounces of boiling water and strain. Dosage: One tablespoon every 3 hours; or:

Tincture of Boneset (*Eupratorium perfoliatum*)	5 to 10 drops
Tincture of Pheasant Eye (*Autumnalis vernalis*)	½ to 2 drops
Tincture of Lady's Slipper (*Cypripedium pubescens*)	5 to 15 drops

In water every 4 hours. Dosage may be reduced or increased according to symptoms. All stimulants must be forbidden. No exertion is permitted.

ERUPTIVE DISEASES

Chicken Pox, Measles, German Measles

Generally palliatives only are necessary, chosen from, or combined: Virginia Snakeroot, Pennyroyal, Catnip, Chamomile, Spearmint. Best given in infusions or teas. Complications must be treated accordingly.

FEVERS

Treatment in General

In almost all instances except in low grade fevers there is a temperature in the beginning, and if this has attention, development may be arrested by elimination and reestablishing a balance.

Of *prime* importance is the Thomsonian course of medication, or another form of relaxing procedure should be followed.

Tincture of Pleurisy Root (*Asclepias tuberose*)	8 to 10 drops
Tincture of Indian Tobacco (*Lobelia inflata*)	3 to 5 drops
Tincture of Catnip (*Nepeta cataria*)	10 to 15 drops

In warm water every 3 or 4 hours. Amount and frequency governed by age and condition. In domestic practice, infusion is best.

Pleurisy Root (*Asclepsias tuberose*)	1 teaspoon
Catnip (*Nepeta cataria*)	1 teaspoon
Indian Tobacco (*Lobelia inflata*)	¼ teaspoon

Steeped in 8 ounces of boiling water for 30 minutes, strain. Adults: 2 tablespoons every hour or according to condition. Children, 1 small tablespoon every hour or according to condition. Always in warm water.

GALL STONES

In many instances it is possible to dissolve formed gall stones, or prevent their formation by proper medication. Formulas that have proven very effective are:

Tincture of Tetterwort (*Sanguinaria canadensis*)	5 to 10 drops
Tincture of Barberry (*Berberis vulgaris*)	3 to 5 drops
Tincture of Fringe Tree (*Chiolanthus virginica*)	3 to 5 drops
Tincture of Bitter Root (*Apocynum Androsaemifolium*)	1 to 2 drops

In water 3 times a day, best one-half hour after meals; or:

Tincture of Wormseed	8 to 10 drops
Tincture of Rheumatism Root (*Dioscores villosa*)	1 to 5 drops
Tincture of Mandrake (*Podophyllum peltatum*)	1 to 3 drops
Tincture of Fringe Tree (*Chiolanthus virginica*)	3 to 5 drops

In water 3 to 4 times a day.

GANGRENE

Morbid Sores and Infections

Four ounces comfrey steeped in 8 ounces of boiling water for 1 hour, strain. Add 4 ounces non-alcoholic Marygold, 2 ounces Coneflower, and 2 ounces Myrrh. Clean diseased part. Fold linen or cotton sheeting 4 to 6 times, wet, and apply with bandages; wet several times a day. Change in the evening. Very effective in the treatment of slow healing ulcers and sores of like nature.

GASTRITIS

Chronic

Tincture of Bayberry (*Myrica cerifera*)	10 to 20 drops
Tincture of Goldenseal (*Hydrastis canadensis*)	10 to 20 drops
Tincture of Fringe Tree (*Chiolanthus virginica*)	5 drops
Tincture of Sweet Flag (*Acorus calamus*)	10 to 20 drops

In 4 ounces of water either before or after meals. In some instances it may be necessary to give it either one-half hour before or after meals. The reaction to the medicine will quickly indicate which is best.

GOITRE

Bronchocele

Goitre, generally a woman's disease, is most frequently associated with irregularity of the menstrual function. This and the general health should receive first attention.

A treatment frequently successful is a combination of iodine, best obtained from the sea weeds and foods rich in this element, and other agents rich in iodine. Consult physician's Armamentarium.

General treatment:

Tincture of Bayberry (*Myrica cerifera*)	8 to 15 drops
Tincture of White Oak Bark (*Quercus alba*)	1 to 5 drops
Tincture of Goldenseal (*Hydrastis canadensis*)	10 to 20 drops

In water 3 to 4 times a day.

Where there is a tendency to overweight, the Natura physician generally prescribes 1 or 2 grains of natural thyroid per day to normalize metabolism.

The diet should be strictly regulated. It should contain very little fats, no sweets of any kind, very few starches, very little salt, and all sea foods. For starches use baked potatoes and brown rice. An abundance of vegetable salads, all green vegetables, and some boiled. There should be no stimulants.

GRAVEL

Tincture of Couch-Grass (*Triticum repens*)	5 to 15 drops
Tincture of Corn Silk (*Stigmata Maydis*)	15 to 30 drops
Tincture of Shave Grass (*Equisetum arvense*)	5 to 20 drops
Tincture of Knotgrass (*Polyganum aviculare*)	15 to 30 drops
Tincture of Hemlock	5 to 15 drops

In 4 ounces of water 3 or 4 times a day.

A very old domestic remedy made into an infusion: One ounce of Corn Silk and Knotgrass. One-half ounce each of Couch-grass,

Shave grass and Hemlock steeped in a quart of boiling water for 30 to 60 minutes, strain. One to 2 tablespoons in water 3 or 4 times a day. The Natura physician usually has best results with the tinctures.

HEADACHE

Bilious

Tincture of Goldenseal (*Hydrastis canadensis*)   8 drops
Tincture of Fringe Tree (*Chiolanthus virginica*)   6 drops
Tincture of Poplar (*Populus tremuloides*)   4 to 8 drops

In water every 3 hours during attack. Three times a day after meals between attacks or as long as necessary.

Bile salts and hydrochloric acid after meals.

Chronic or Stomach

Tincture of Evening Primrose (*Oenothera biennis*)   8 to 15 drops
Tincture of Motherwort (*Leonurus cardiaca*)   8 to 10 drops
Tincture of Goldenseal (*Hydrastis canadensis*)   8 to 10 drops

In water after meals.

Nervous

Tincture of Lady's Slipper (*Cypripedium pubescens*)   8 to 15 drops
Tincture of Pasque Flower (*Anenome pulsatilla*)   1 to 3 drops
Tincture of Passion Flower (*Passiflora incarnata*)   8 to 15 drops

In water every 3 hours during attacks. Twice a day thereafter.

Menstrual

Tincture of Pasque Flower (*Anenome pulsatilla*)   1 to 3 drops
Tincture of Squaw Vine (*Mitchella repens*)   8 to 15 drops
Tincture of Motherwort (*Leonurus cardiaca*)   8 to 15 drops

With water every 3 hours during attack. Three times a day thereafter, as long as necessary.

Heart—(Non-Organic Heart Weakness)

Tincture of Cactus (*Cereus grandiflorus*)   2 to 4 drops
Tincture of Hawthorn (*Crataegus oxyacantha*)   5 to 10 drops

In water 3 or more times a day as long as required, or :

Tincture of Scullcap (*Scutellaria lateriflora*)	8 to 15 drops
Tincture of Hawthorn (*Crataegus oxyacantha*)	4 to 8 drops

With water 3 or more times a day as long as required.

HYPERTENSION—HIGH BLOOD PRESSURE, HARDENING OF THE ARTERIES—ARTERIOSCLEROSIS

Are these different ailments, or *different expressions* (symptoms) *of one condition?*

Is the actual cause known and do the practitioners of any of the schools of medical practice agree on the cause? Is there a cure? This condition, so serious, so universal, is a controversial subject and, therefore has no place in a text of this nature. But because of its seriousness and universality, the Natura physician *must* give it serious thought and investigation; and if possible, find the means to alleviate, if not cure, those so afflicted, who consult him for relief.

Most physicians admit that the present forms of medication cannot cure and, in general, are even valueless to give relief. Serious thinkers have returned to the investigation of the virtues and value of vital elements made use of in the earlier systematized medical practice —the barks and roots of herbs and the vital elements present in the vegetables, flowers, shrubs and even grasses; as an example oat beards for its vital element.

A late example is the use of *Rauwolfia serpentia,* (more generally known as Snakeroot), a plant found in India. It is used in the treatment of high blood pressure. This was publicized by CIBA Pharmaceutical Products when they announced they had isolated that part of *Rauwolfia* which lowers high blood pressure. This is not to be considered as a "cure" for the condition, but a relief. As far as known it has not been tested in preventing the development of high blood pressure and associated conditions, or stopping the development if started and eliminating the cause.

The Snakeroot obtained from India is *not to be confused* with Virginia Snakeroot and its active element Aristollochine which we have found of value combined with other agents in preventing the development of hypertensive—high blood pressure—arteriosclerosis, because of its effectiveness in stomach ailments, basing its use on the theory that these conditions have their beginning in interference with digestion, malassimilation and elimination, unless caused by other diseases.

It is generally believed that one of two things cause hardening of the arteries or arteriosclerosis. It is due either to fats, or sugars and starches. We (speaking for ourselves personally) based our investigation on the concept that *both* were *causative* of this condition.

Consider first fats as the cause. Why? How? Our thought reverted to our grandmothers, even mother, making soap. To do this, they saved all their fats, then with the addition of an alkali (usually soot from the chimney), they *boiled* this into soap. If an *insufficient* amount of some form of potash was added, they failed. The system does, or should do, this very thing. It employs bile to saponify the fats. If we believe there is an insufficient amount of bile to do this, the conversion of the fat is incomplete; it cannot be properly absorbed. It creates effete matter, which clogs the system and interferes with the circulation, gradually doing to the veins what lime and iron in water do to water pipes. In like manner, if sugars and starches are not turned into natural alcohol, the same thing takes place.

Accepting this theory, we began our experimenting with the thought that, as already stated, digestion, assimilation, and elimination must have attention. First consideration always being given to the first symptoms of hypertension by a careful and complete checkup. If no signs of other causative conditions, then it must be concluded that the physical agents which alone can fully convert fats, sugar, and starches are insufficient to bring about this conversion and prevent the creation of foreign, *effete matter which changes into cholesterol.*

Having in mind the old manner of making soap and the need of a converter of fats, our conclusion was that the lack of digestive agents and bile was the primary cause, and therefore a substitute must be found. This was not difficult, because in the past, (before modern chemical agents were substituted for organic agents such as tinctures), fluid extracts and powders were in universal use.

Our formulas consisted and still consist in variation, of:

Tincture of Oregon Grape (*Berberis aquifolium*)	10 to 20 drops
Tincture of Barberry (*Berberis vulgaris*)	5 to 10 drops
Tincture of Goldenseal (*Hydrastis canadensis*)	8 to 10 drops
Tincture of Mandrake (*Podophyllum peltatum*)	Sufficient for proper elimination.

In water after meals ; or :

Tincture of Goldenseal (*Hydrastis canadensis*)	8 to 10 drops
Tincture of Fringe Tree (*Chiolanthus virginica*)	7 to 10 drops
Tincture of Yellow Gentian Root (*Gentiana lutea*)	5 to 20 drops
Tincture of Oregon Grape (*Berberis aquifolium*)	10 to 20 drops
Tincture of Mandrake (*Podophyllum peltata*)	sufficient for

proper elimination, and/or, bile salts in conjunction with these formulas.

In water after meals.

Intake of salt should be radically reduced. Fats with exception of milk, some cream, and a small amount of butter eliminated. Sugars and starches are prohibited. Sea food and protein predominating. Plenty of fresh vegetables in every form. Brown rice and baked potatoes substituting for other starches.

This procedure is usually effective in at first retarding then eliminating the condition, (if not due to other diseases) and started at the beginning of the condition.

HYSTERIA

Female Disturbances

Tincture of Lady's Slipper (*Cypripedium pubescens*)	8 to 15 drops
Tincture of Motherwort (*Leonurus cardiaca*)	10 to 15 drops
Tincture of Pasque Flower (*Anenome pulsatilla*)	1 to 3 drops
Tincture of Scullcap (*Scutellaria lateriflora*)	8 to 15 drops

In water every hour during attacks.

INDIGESTION

Acute

Tincture of Poplar (*Populus tremuloides*)	3 to 6 drops
Tincture of Fringe Tree (*Chiolanthus virginica*)	5 to 9 drops
Tincture of Goldenseal (*Hydrastis canadensis*)	7 to 10 drops
Tincture of Bitter Root (*Apocynum Androsaemifolium*)	3 to 5 drops

In water after meals or during attacks.

Atonic

Tincture of Goldenseal (*Hydrastis canadensis*)	7 to 10 drops
Tincture of Yellow Gentian Root (*Gentiana lutea*)	10 to 15 drops
Tincture of St. John's Wort (*Hypericum perforatum*)	5 to 10 drops
Tincture of Cayenne Pepper (*Capsicum frutescens*)	8 drops

In water after meals.

Flatulence of Wind Colic

Tincture of Sweet Flag (*Acorus Calamus*)	10 to 15 drops
Tincture of Feverfew (*Chrysanthemum Parthenium*)	10 drops
Tincture of Peppermint (*Mentha piperta*)	8 to 12 drops
Tincture of Spearmint (*Mentha viridis*)	5 to 8 drops

In water during attacks as necessary.

Intestinal

Tincture of Goldenseal (*Hydrastis canadensis*)	8 drops
Tincture of Yellow Gentian Root (*Gentiana lutea*)	10 to 15 drops

In water after meals.

INSOMNIA

Tincture of Peach Leaves (*Prunus Persica*)	4 to 10 drops
Tincture of Passion Flower (*Passiflora incarnata*)	5 to 10 drops
Tincture of Lady's Slipper (*Cypripedium pubescens*)	3 to 10 drops
Tincture of Scullcap (*Scutellaria lateriflora*)	3 to 15 drops

Dosage and frequency governed by age and symptoms; or:

Tincture of Lady's Slipper (*Cypripedium pubescens*)	3 to 15 drops
Tincture of Chamomile (*Anthemis nobilis*)	10 to 20 drops
Tincture of Passion Flower (*Passiflora incaraata*)	5 to 10 drops

Dosage and frequency governed by age and symptoms.

In using this prescription it is best, when possible, to separate the Chamomile from the rest of the formula making an infusion of 1 teaspoon of the herb in a cup of boiling water for one-half hour; strain. 1 tablespoon in water 4 times a day and a cup before retiring. The tinctures, 3 or more times a day.

JAUNDICE

Icterus

Tincture of Bitter Root (*Apocynum Androsaemifolium*)	10 to 20 drops
Tincture of Cascara Sagrada (*Phamnus purshianus*)	10 to 20 drops
Tincture of Ginger (*Zingiber officinale*)	10 to 15 drops

Dosage: 3 times a day, preferably after meals, according to condition. Amount of Cascara only sufficient for proper elimination. No stimulants or fatty foods allowed. Diet should be simple.

Or:

Tincture of Yellow Gentian (*Gentiana lutea*)	15 to 30 drops
Tincture of Fringe Tree (*Chiolanthus virginica*)	5 to 10 drops
Tincture of Bitter Root (*Apocynum Androsaemifolium*)	1 to 3 drops
Tincture of Mandrake (*Podophyllum peltatum*)	2 to 4 drops

Dosage according to condition.

Only sufficient Mandrake should be included in the formula necessary for regular and sufficient elimination.

Or:

Tincture of Poplar (*Populus tremuloides*)	4 to 8 drops
Tincture of Bitter Root (*Apocynum Androsaemifolium*)	4 to 10 drops
Tincture of Feverfew (*Chrysanthemum Parthenium*)	10 to 15 drops
Tincture of Rhubarb	5 to 20 drops

Dosage according to symptoms, 3 to 4 times a day.

Only sufficient Rhubarb should be added to the formula for regular and sufficient elimination.

KIDNEY INFLAMMATION—ACUTE

Nephritis

Acute nephritis should be considered as an emergency disease and treated accordingly. Consult physician's Armamentarium. General treatment when there is a temperature:

Tincture of Pleurisy Root (*Asclepias tuberose*)	15 to 30 drops
Tincture of Marsh Mallow (*Althea officinalis*)	10 to 20 drops

Preferable in warm water.

Domestically, an infusion of 2 ounces each of Pleurisy Root and Marsh Mallow steeped in a pint of boiling water for one-half hour. Two tablespoons every 2 hours has been very successful.

Tincture of Shepherd's Purse (*Capsella bursapastoris*)	15 to 30 drops
Tincture of Peach Tree Leaves (*Prunus Persica*)	10 to 20 drops
Tincture of Hollyhock (*Althea rosea*)	10 to 30 drops

In water every 2 to 3 hours.

If there is blood in the urine, add:

Tincture of Witch Hazel (*Hamamelis virginiana*)	15 to 30 drops
Tincture of Myrrh (*Commiphora myrrha*)	2 drops

KIDNEYS

Mucus in Urine

Tincture of Motherwort (*Leonurus cardiaca*)	8 to 20 drops
Tincture of Linden Flowers (*Tillis Europaea*)	10 to 20 drops
Tincture of Couch-Grass (*Triticum repens*)	20 to 40 drops
Tincture of Shave Grass (*Equisetum arvense*)	13 to 30 drops

In water 3 or 4 times a day.

LA GRIPPE

Frequently called Influenza

Tincture of Pleurisy Root (*Asclepias tuberose*)	10 drops
Tincture of Boneset (*Eupatorium perfoliatum*)	15 drops
Tincture of Scullcap (*Scutellaria latriflora*)	8 drops

Dosage according to age and symptoms, always in warm water every 3 hours or more. When chills are present, 3 drops of Cayenne Pepper should be added. If relaxing is indicated 4 to 8 drops of Indian Tobacco.

For infusion, 1 teaspoon of Pleurisy root and Boneset, three-quarters teaspoon Scullcap steeped in 8 ounces boiling water for one-half hour. Strain. 1 tablespoon in hot water every 3 or 4 hours. Give to children proportionately.

LEUCORRHOEA

Persistent

Tincture of Cranesbill (*Geranium Maculatum*)	5 to 20 drops
Tincture of White Pond Lily Root (*Nymphaea odorata*)	5 to 20 drops
Tincture of Marigold (*Calendula officinalis*)	8 to 15 drops
Tincture of Pasque Flower (*Anenome pulsatilla*)	2 drops

In water 3 or 4 times a day.

If there is odor or pus, add 2 drops of Myrrh.

Tincture of Pipsissewa (*Chimaphila umbellata*)	8 to 15 drops

Other indicated remedies according to condition: Bayberry, Bearberry, Sumach, Witch-Hazel, Red Raspberry and Tormemtil.

LIVER

Cirrhosis

Cirrhosis of the liver is generally the result of abuses such as excessive use of alcohol, sweets of every description, or other dietary abuses. To effect relief or a cure *drastic* steps must be taken to eliminate these abuses.

Cirrhosis may also be the result or associated with various other diseases, and these must receive proper treatment.

A general treatment that has proven effective:

Tincture of Goldenseal (*Hydrastis canadensis*)	8 to 10 drops
Tincture of Fringe Tree (*Chiolanthus virginica*)	4 to 8 drops
Tincture of Yellow Gentian (*Gentiana lutea*)	5 to 8 drops
Tincture of Cascara Sagrada (*Rhamnus purshianus*)	Sufficient
	amount for proper elimination.

In water after each meal.

In many cases it is advisable to include bile salts.

Spleen Involvement

Tincture of Jersey Tea (*Ceanthus americanus*)	10 to 20 drops
Tincture of Fringe Tree (*Chiolanthus virginica*)	5 to 10 drops
Tincture of Barberry (*Berberis vulgaris*)	10 to 20 drops
Tincture of Goldenseal (*Hydrastis canadensis*)	5 to 10 drops

In water before meals.

Engorgement

Tincture of Dandelion	20 to 40 drops
Tincture of Bitter Root (*Apocynum Androsaemifolium*)	3 to 7 drops
Tincture of Goldenseal (*Hydrastis canadensis*)	5 to 10 drops

In water after meals.

Bile salts and hydrochloric acid frequently indicated.

Inflammation—Acute

Tincture of Fringe Tree (*Chiolanthus virginica*)	5 to 8 drops
Tincture of Jersey Tea (*Ceanthus americanus*)	10 to 20 drops
Tincture of Bitter Root (*Apocynum Androsaemifolium*)	3 to 7 drops

In water after meals. All fats and sweets in any form are prohibited and very little salt permitted.

Torpid

Tincture of Barberry (*Berberis vulgaris*)	8 to 15 drops
Tincture of Yellow Gentian Root (*Gentiana lutea*)	3 to 10 drops
Tincture of Bitter Wood	3 to 15 drops
Tincture of Goldenseal (*Hydrastis canadensis*)	5 to 10 drops

MALARIA

Tincture of Pleurisy Root (*Asclepias tuberose*)	7 to 12 drops
Tincture of Barberry (*Berberis vulgaris*)	8 to 15 drops
Tincture of Peruvian Bark (*Cinchona succirubra*)	2 drops
Tincture of Cayenne Pepper (*Capsicum frutescens*)	2 drops

In hot water every 2 to 4 hours according to symptoms. *Not* to be prescribed for pregnant women.

MARASMUS

Malnutrition

A condition generally resulting from a diet deficient in necessary nutriment, chiefly proper protein and mineral elements. Treatment must be first, to supply the missing elements, then to stimulate appetite, digestion, and assimulation.

Tincture of Goldenseal (*Hydrastis canadensis*)	5 to 10 drops
Tincture of Fringe Tree (*Chiolanthus virginica*)	3 to 8 drops
Tincture of Bitter Root	3 to 10 drops

In water 3 or 4 times a day.

All sweets and fats are prohibited. Baked potatoes, brown rice, barley, and okra should be substituted for all starches. No tea, coffee, or stimulants (herb teas substituted). Bile salts included in remedies for elimination.

MELANCHOLY

Associated with Various Diseases

Melancholy, neurasthenia, and neurosis are seldom diseases in themselves but are associated with various ailments and diseases and require medical attention. They are seldom curable unless the disease they are associated with is treated and eliminated.

Tincture of Lady's Slipper (*Cypripedium pubescens*)	10 to 20 drops
Titncure of Jersey Tea (*Ceanthus americanus*)	3 to 15 drops
Tincture of Motherwort (*Leonurus cardiaca*)	15 to 30 drops
Tincture of Pasque Flower (*Anenome pulsatilla*)	2 to 4 drops

In water 3 or 4 times a day.

MENSTRUAL IRREGULARITIES

Tincture of Cranesbill (*Geranium Malculatum*)	10 to 20 drops
Tincture of Pennyroyal (*Mentha pulegium*)	10 to 20 drops
Tincture of Tansy (*Tanacetum vulgare*)	2 to 8 drops
Tincture of Chamomile (*Anthemia nobilis*)	13 to 30 drops
Tincture of Pasque Flower (*Anenome pulsatilla*)	1 to 3 drops

In water 3 or 4 times a day as required.

NERVOUSNESS

Nervines

There are numerous types of nervousness for which no apparent cause can be found; and diagnosis is most difficult. Those who do suffer one form or another are generally miserable and in need of natural agents totally unharmful to the system, yet are highly successful sedatives and should be prescribed. In many instances there have been household remedies, though not reasonably prescribed or well combined. This can be readily corrected:

Tincture of Scullcap (*Scutellaria lateriflora*)	2 to 15 drops
Tincture of Lady's Slipper (*Cypripedium pubescens*)	5 to 10 drops
Tincture of Passion Flower (*Passiflora incarnata*)	10 to 20 drops

In water several times a day and before retiring.

Or:

Tincture of Scullcap (*Scutellaria lateriflora*)	2 to 15 drops
Tincture of Lady's Slipper (*Cypripedium pubescens*)	15 to 30 drops
Tincture of Passion Flower (*Passiflora incarnata*)	10 to 30 drops

In water as required and before retiring.

In nervousness during menses and menopause, add 2 to 5 drops tincture of Pasque Flower.

NEURALGIA

Female

Tincture of Bitter Root (*Apocynum Androsaemifolium*)	4 to 8 drops
Tincture of Lady's Slipper (*Cypripedium pubescens*)	5 to 10 drops
Tincture of Pasque Flower (*Anenome pulsatilla*)	2 to 4 drops

In water every 3 to 4 hours during attack.

Bitter Root, although a valuable agent, should, like Pasque Flower be given only in very small doses.

NEURITIS

Tincture of Bitter Root (*Apocynum Androsaemifolium*)	4 to 8 drops
Tincture of Motherwort (*Leonurus cardiaca*)	10 to 20 drops
Tincture of Lady's Slipper (*Cypripedium pubescens*)	10 to 20 drops

In water every 3 to 4 hours during attack.

PERITONITIS

An emergency condition. To be treated according to symptoms. Generally, first choice, the Thomsonian procedure. Secondly:

Tincture of Coneflower (*Echinaces angustifolia*)	15 to 40 drops
Tincture of Wild Indigo (*Baptista tinctoria*)	2 drops
Tincture of Myrrh (*Commiphora myrrha*)	2 drops

With other medication in warm water.

PLEURISY

Tincture of Pleurisy Root (*Asclepias tuberose*)	10 to 15 drops
Tincture of Scullcap (*Scutellaria lateriflora*)	8 to 10 drops
Tincture of Boneset (*Eupatorium perfoliatum*)	15 drops

In warm water every 2 to 4 hours according to symptoms.

Ginger and Pennyroyal tea as a liquid.

In domestic practice, 1 teaspoon of the herbs steeped in 8 ounces of boiling water for 30 minutes, strain. One to 2 tablespoons in warm water every 2 to 4 hours.

PNEUMONIA

Pneumonia must be considered as an emergency condition. General treatment:

Tincture of Scullcap (*Scutellaria lateriflora*)	8 to 10 drops
Tincture of Boneset (*Boneset perifoliatum*)	8 to 15 drops
Tincture of Pleurisy Root (*Asclepias tuberose*)	7 to 10 drops
Tincture of Feverfew (*Chrysanthemum parthenium*)	10 to 15 drops

In warm water every 2 or 3 hours.

If symptoms indicate:

Tincture of Motherwort (*Leonurus cardiaca*)	15 to 30 drops

Between other medication, warm Pennyroyal and Ginger tea as liquids.

PROSTATITIS
Non-Operative

Tincture of Saw Palmetto	10 to 20 drops
Tincture of Couch-Grass (*Triticum repens*)	5 to 15 drops
Tincture of Pipsissewa (*Chimaphila umbellata*)	2 to 10 drops
Tincture of Pasque Flower (*Anenome pulsatilla*)	2 to 4 drops

In water 4 times a day.

PUERPERAL FEVER

Like typhoid and scarlet fever it is to be considered an emergency condition because of its seriousness and the possibility of complications.

General treatment:

Tincture of Coneflower (*Echinacea angustifolia*)	15 to 40 drops
Tincture of Wild Indigo (*Baptista tinctoria*)	2 drops
Tincture of Feverfew (*Chrysanthemum parthenium*)	10 to 20 drops
Tincture of Myrrh (*Commiphora myrrha*)	2 drops

Every 2 to 4 hours. Passion Flower together with Catnip, Pennyroyal or other soothing teas for restlessness.

RHEUMATISM

General

Tincture of Black Cohash (*Cimicifuga racemosa*)	2 to 10 drops
Tincture of Pipsissewa (*Chimaphila umbellata*)	2 to 10 drops
Tincture of Bitter Root (*Apocynum Androsaemifolium*)	2 to 8 drops
Tincture of Motherwort (*Leonurus cardiaca*)	10 to 20 drops
Tincture of Evening Primrose (*Oenathe biennis*)	5 to 10 drops

In water 4 times a day.

SCARLET FEVER

Considered an emergency condition because of the care essential to avoid complications. General treatment for fevers to be followed. Complications to be treated accordingly. Quiet, darkened room, no disturbances. Ginger, Pennyroyal, and Catnip teas for liquids; Passion Flower for restlessness. Elimination is important. Refer to agents under physician's Armamentarium.

SINUSITIS—RHINITIS

These conditions, now so general, persistent, and discouraging to the sufferer, should not be considered as a disease, but an ailment due to many causes that should be sought and properly treated.

Most generally, the basic cause is to be found in the diet, poor sanitary conditions, and inadequate elimination. This must be corrected if the condition is to be overcome and eliminated. Medication must be consistent, otherwise, the symptoms may become chronic.

Tincture of Tetterwort (*Sanguiniara canadensis*)	8 to 10 drops
Tincture of Pasque Flower (*Anenome pulsatilla*)	1 to 2 drops
Tincture of Mandrake (*Polophyllum peltatum*)	¼ to 5 drops
Tincture of Evening Primrose (*Oenathea biennia*)	5 to 10 drops

In water 3 or 4 times a day.

SMALLPOX

To be treated in like matter as scarlet fever. Elimination to receive careful attention. Quiet, dark room; complications treated accordingly.

In all morbid conditions the Thomsonian plan of treatment is generally effective. Consult physician's Armamentarium.

STOMACH

Bitters—Stimulants to Digestion

Tincture of Yellow Gentian (*Gentiana lutea*)	10 to 20 drops
Tincture of Goldenseal (*Hydrastis canadensis*)	6 to 10 drops
Tincture of Chamomile (*Anthemis nobilis*)	12 to 20 drops
Tincture of Oregon Grape (*Berberis aquifolium*)	5 to 10 drops

In water before meals.

TYPHOID FEVER

This must be considered an emergency condition. General treatment with variation:

Tincture of Cranesbill (*Geranium Maculatum*)	20 to 50 drops
Tincture of Wild Indigo (*Baptista tinctoria*)	2 drops
Tincture of Coneflower (*Echinaces angustifolia*)	15 to 40 drops
Tincture of Bayberry (*Myrica Cerifera*)	20 to 40 drops

Every 3 to 4 hours in water. Passion Flower for nerve tension or restlessness.

ULCERS

Gastric

Tincture of Goldenseal (*Hydrastis canadensis*)	6 to 10 drops
Tincture of Carolina Jasmine	1 to 4 drops
Tincture of Coneflower (*Echinacea angustifolia*)	10 to 20 drops
Tincture of Pleurisy root (*Asclepias tuberose*)	1 to 10 drops

In water after meals.

Gastric ulcers are generally caused by a faulty diet—fats, starches, sugars, salt, and stimulants, especially alcoholic beverages. All these must be curtailed, if not entirely eliminated. A bland diet should be substituted, if a cure is expected.

URINE DIFFICULTIES

Incontinence and Scaldy

Tincture of Couch-Grass (*Triticum repens*)	5 to to 10 drops
Tincture of Sumach (*Rhus glabra*)	10 to 20 drops
Tincture of Buchu (*Barosma belulina*)	2 to 10 drops
Tincture of Clivers (*Galium aparine*)	10 to 20 drops

In water 4 times a day.

Scanty and Irritating

Tincture of Corn Silk (*Stigmata Maydis*)	12 to 25 drops
Tincture of Pipsissewa (*Chimaphila umbellata*)	2 to 15 drops
Tincture of Poplar (*Populus tremuloides*)	10 to 20 drops
Tincture of Shave Grass (*Equisetum arvense*)	15 to 25 drops

UTERINE

Tampon Dressing

Tincture of Marigold (*Calendula officinalis*)	10 drops
Tincture of White Pond Lily (*Nymphaea odorata*)	5 drops
Tincture of Bayberry	5 drops
Tincture of Cranesbill (*Geranium Maculatum*)	3 drops

One tampon inserted at night (lying on back and pushing easily up uterus as far as possible). If much mucus, blood, or odor, add 2 drops of tincture of Myrrh. Remove in the morning; follow by douche to which is added Witch-Hazel.

Before following this procedure, there should be a careful examination to learn whether there is a malignancy.

ADDENDUM

To repeat a law of the *beginnings*:[1]

"And God said, Behold, I have given you every herb bearing seed, which is upon the face of all the earth, and every tree, in which is the fruit of a tree yielding seed; *to you* it shall be for meat (food).

"And to every beast of the earth, and to every fowl of the air, and to everything that creepeth upon the earth, wherein there is life, I have given green herb for meat: and it was so."—*Genesis 1:29, 30*.

This statement, a Law given by the Divine to His creatures, has always been accepted *as a basic truth* by every Thomsonian, physio-medical, and *Natura* physician, and has governed their practice though generally used in the form of a tincture or fluid extract.

The herbs of the fields and woodland and their seeds are *actually foods* for the body and mind. They contain vital elements such as vitamins and minerals, even as do those articles of sustenance we usually class as foods. *In addition, they contain active principles* which act as agents (medicines) to heal the wounds of the body or eliminate destructive poisons from the system.

Some of these herbs are classified as poisonous or narcotics. An example is *Cannabis Indica*[2] or Indian hemp. It is doubtful if there is a single chemical compound as effective in the treatment of various forms of ailments under the classification of "neurosis" when properly prescribed.

Paolo Rovesti and Bianco Magno of Milan, Italy by experimentation with yellow corn sprouts have found that the extracts contain vitamins, organic minerals, an antibiotic (organic) and an antioxidant (organic).[3]

---

1. This statement is extremely pertinent in view of the latest discoveries by men of science who have been experimenting with the vital, or active principles in various seeds.

2. Admittedly this is a poison, but there is probably no substance that is not destructive in too great an amount. Even water, a substance the body must be supplied with daily to properly function, in too great an amount may be causative of disease.

3. We are taking pains to mention that these substances are *organic* because the system can metabolize them as food while we do not believe it can the *inorganics*.

These scientists have also found that the juice of wheat contains vitamin E. Every experienced dietician has long been aware of this. In barley juice they have found vitamin B¹ so essential in preventing and curing diseases of the nature of beriberi. They have found that such seeds also contain vitamin C and niacin, which they class as a preventive of diseases of the nature of pellagra.

Another scientist, Peter A. Ark, professor of plant pathology in the University of California at Berkeley, has found that wheat and barley extracts contain antibiotic substances important in the treatment of germ and fungi diseases.

In India at the Dacca University, Drs. H. N. De and S. C. Datta have found that in the germinated or sprouted seeds of legumes and grains grown in India, such as cowpeas, peas, rice, and the grains especially wheat and barley, niacin is found in considerable quantities.[4]

Scientists Baude, Kon, Mitchell, and Kodiceh of the University of Reading, England, have been able to demonstrate that niacin is associated with other properties of great medicinal and nutritional value in almost all seeds, hence in their sprouts eaten as salads.

In the treatment of stomach and intestinal ulcers, dieticians have found that barley soaked in warm (not hot) water for from 8 to 10 hours and this water consumed as would be ordinary water, possesses a powerful neutralizing influence on irritating acids frequently causative of ulcers. The barley, then cooked with vegetables, including much okra, which also possesses neutralizing, healing substances.

Russian scientists, associated with the Academy of Science, Moscow, have found that sunflower, wheat, barley, and soybeans are not only rich in niacin, but also in vitamin B¹ and riboflavin essential in the growth of children, and in the prevention of cataract and diseases of the skin. Fresh sprouts of these seeds are of greater value than the extracts or processed products.

Penicillin has proven extremely valuable in many diseased conditions, but at the same time is a dangerous remedy to many people. Biblically speaking, there is an *organic* penicillin which may be extracted from the ash, pivit, rose, acaci, and honey locust seeds.

---

4. In view of the fact that almost all grain foods are denuded of their vital elements in their processing, the experienced dietician and *Natura* physician now strongly advocates the sprouting of the various seeds, especially such as mung beans, alfalfa seeds, soybeans, oats (rich in Avena sativa) and wheat, making them into salads wth their meals daily.

To refer again to foods, the scientists Pievo Gallo and Humberto Valeri have found that the delicious, and much enjoyed, avocado pear is rich in antibiotic substances.

Scientist V. A. Skovronskii of Russia has found that the seed of the common caraway, ains, and sweet fennel contain substances of great value as a diuretic in the treatment of swellings and the accumulation of fluids in the body when due to various heart, lung and kidney diseases.

Much is said of the extensive use of dangerous tranquilizers. Is there such a thing as a *natural,* i.e., *organic* tranquilizer? Scientists Argawal Dandiya and associates in a medical College in Jaipur, India have found that the extracts from carrots[5] are relaxants of the muscles and intestines as well as the nervous system and of value in obstetrics where there is tenseness.

The Thomsonian, physio-medical and *Natura* schools of medicines are all closed and only a small number of the practitioners of these systems survive. This is most regrettable now that these natural remedies are coming into favor once again and may replace the great number of complicated chemical compounds many of which have proved to be highly dangerous in practice. The Lord's words of times beyond counting: "Behold I have given you every herb bearing seed, etc." is slowly being verified by scientists.

---

5. A great amount of carrot juice is consumed by those believing they are following a natural diet. This juice is of great value to the system if taken in proper proportion of possibly no more than 4 ounces a day. Greater amounts may be as destructive to the liver as the excessive use of alcoholics. *Temperance* is the Law in all things.

CLINICAL INDEX

To simplify the selection of any agent for a given purpose, we give both the common name and the one known in medical nomenclature. Under the heading of the various ailments we give only the name by which the agent is most generally known to the layman.

COMMON NAME	*LATIN*
Lobelia (Indian Tobacco)	*Lobelia inflata*
Capiscum (Red Pepper)	*Capsicum fastigiatum*
Goldenseal	*Hydrastis canadensis*
Bayberry	*Myrica cerifera*
Chamomile	*Anthemis nobilis* and *Matricara Chamomilla*
Black Samson	*Echinacea angustifolia*
Myrrh	*Balsamodendron myrrha*
Ladyslipper or Valerian	*Cypripedium pubescence*
Crowfoot	*Geranium mac.*
Male Fern (Malefern)	*Aspidium filix-mas*
Gentian	*Gentiana lutae*
Bitterherb or Balmony	*Chelone glabra*
Fringe Tree	*Chionanthus virginica*
Barberry	*Berberis vulgaris*
Passion Flower	*Passiflora incarnata*
Pleurisy Root	*Asclepias tuberosa*
Scullcap	*Scutellaria lateriflora*
Motherwort	*Leonurus cardiaca*
Red Root or Jersey Tea	*Ceanothus Americanus*
Couch Grass	*Triticum repens*
Corn Silk	*Stigmata maydis*
Squaw Vine	*Mitchella repens*
Feverfew	*Chrysanthemum parthenium*
May Flower (Mayflower)	*Pulsatilla nigra*
Poplar Bark	*Populus tremuloides*

COMMON NAME	LATIN
Bearberry	*Uva ursi*
Pipsissewa	*Chimaphila umbellata*
Ginger	*Zingiber*
Pond Lily	*Nymphaea odorata*
Hemlock	*Canadensis*
Sumach (Sumac)	*Rhus glabra*
Witch-Hazel (Wichhazel)	*Hamamelis virginiana*
Red Raspberry	*Rubus strigosus*
Bitter Root (Bitterroot) or Milk Weed	*Apocynum androsaemifolium*
Pennyroyal	*Hedeoma pulegioides*
Hoarhound or Horehound	*Marrubium vulgare*
Spearmint	*Mentha viridis*
Peppermint	*Mentha piperita*
Tansy	*Tanacetum vulgare*
Bitter Sweet (Bittersweet)	*Solanum dulcamara*
Burdock	*Actium lappa*
Yellow Dock (Yellowdock)	*Rumex crispus*
Dandelion	*Leontodon taraxacum*
Virginia Snakeroot	*Aristolochia serpentaria*
Buchu	*Barosma betulina*
Cleavers or Clivers	*Qualium aparine*
Black Currant Leaves	*Ribes nigrum*
Blueberries	*Vaccinium myrtillus*
Coltsfoot	*Tussilago farfara*
Dwarf Elder	*Sambucus ebulus* and *Aralia hispida*
Eyebright	*Euphrasia officinalis*
Fennel	*Foeniculum officinalis*
Knot Grass	*Polygonum aviculare*
Linden Flowers	*Tilia Europaea*
Mallow Flowers	*Althea rosea*
Marigold Flowers	*Calendula officinalis*
Milkwort	*Polygala vulgaris*
Mullein Flowers	*Varbascum thapsus*
Oak Bark	*Quercus rubur*

COMMON NAME	LATIN
Oat Beards	*Avena sativa*
Primrose	*Primula officinalis*
Rosemary	*Rosmarinus officinalis*
St. John's Wort	*Hypericum perforatum*
Sage	*Salvia officinalis*
Scurvy Grass	*Cochlearia officinalis*
Silverweed	*Potentilla anserina*
Strawberry leaves	*Fragaria vesca*
Sweet-Flag	*Acorus calamus*
Tormentil	*Potentilla tormentilla*
Vervain Root	*Verbena officinalis*
Violet	*Viola odorata*
Watercress	*Nasturtium officinalis*
Flaxseed	*Linum usitatissimum*

Abscesses

Chamomile

Acidosis

Motherwort   Charcoal   Watercress   Calamus

Albumen and Phosphates in Urine

Motherwort   Corn Silk

Anemia

Bayberry   *Pulsatilla   Myrica   Hydrasis   Oats*
Capsicum

Asthma

Lobelia   Passiflora   Pulsatilla   Myrrh   Hoarhound

Enuresis (bed-wetting)

Calendula   St. John's Wort   Mullein

Blood Poisoning

Echinacea

Brick Dust in Urine

Corn Silk

Bronchitis

Feverfew   *Lobelia*

Bronchitis (Chronic)

Hydrasis   Geranium   Mullein flowers   Hoarhound
Linden leaves   Myrrh   *Ceanothus*

Burns

Calendula   Vaseline

Catarrh (Bronchial)

Barberry

Catarrh (Foul mucus)

Hydrastis   Barberry   *Myrica   Echinacea*   Hoarhound
Black Currant Leaves   *Lobelia*

Catarrh (Nasal)

Calendula   Hydrastis   Mullein flowers   Linden leaves

Childbirth, Made Easy

Squaw vine

Cholera Infantum

Geranium   Hydrastis   Barberry   Poplar Bark
Dewberry

Coffee (Tonic)

Acorns   Oats

Colds (Acute)

Pleurisy root   Boneset   Ginger   Pennyroyal   Hoarhound
Peppermint   Rosemary

Colds (deep seated)

Myrrh

Colic (Bilious)

Chionanthus   Lobelia

Colic in Children

Chamomile   Ginger   Pennyroyal   Spearmint
Peppermint   Fennel

Constipation

Rhubarb   Licorice   Bitter root   Dandelion
Aloes   *Hydrastis*

Consumption

Myrrh   *Ceanothus   Capsicum   Hydrastis*

Convalescence and Debility

Barberry   *Hydrastis   Capsicum*   Gentian   Bitter Herb
Acorns   Oats

Convulsions in Infants

Bitter-Sweet

Cough (Chronic with Phlegm)

Coltsfoot   Linden Flowers   Hoarhound

Cough (Whooping)

Black Currant Leaves   Vervain Root   Violet   *Ceanothus*

Deafness

Mullein

Delirium

Cypripedium

Delirium Tremens

Motherwort   *Passiflora*   *Cypripedium*

Dementia in Change of Life

Cypripedium

Diabetes

Bearberry   Buchu   Blueberries

Diarrhoea (Acute)

Geranium   *Hydrastis*   Bayberry   Myrrh   *Pulsatilla*
Poplar Bark   Bearberry   White Pond Lily   Hemlock
Sumac   Witch Hazel   Red Raspberry   Dewberry
Blueberries

Diarrhoea (Acid)

Chamomile

Diarrhoea (Chronic)

Myrrh   Poplar Bark   Bearberry   White Pond Lily
Echinacea

Diarrhoea (Summer)

Dewberry   Witch-Hazel   Rhubarb   *Echinacea*

Diarrhoea (Scrofulus)

Bayberry   White Pond Lily

Diphtheria

Lobelia   *Echinacea*   Myrrh

Dyspepsia (Acute)

Chionanthus

Dropsy

Myrrh   Pipsissewa   Poplar Bark   Dandelion   Dwarf Elder
Scurvy Grass   Rosemary

Dropsy, due to faulty liver

Bitter Herb   Dandelion

Dysentery

Geranium   Bayberry   *Ceanothus*   Poplar Bark   Witch Hazel
Red Raspberry   Dewberry

Dysentery, during pregnancy

Squaw Vine   Dewberry   Red Raspberry

Dyspepsia

Hydrastis   Gentian   Bitter herb   Bonset   Bitter root
Oak Bark   St. John's Wort

Dyspepsia (Atonic)

Bitter Herb   *Hydrastis*   Poplar Bark   Gentian
Berberis   Myrrh

Dyspepsia (Chronic)

Rumex   Bayberry

Dyspepsia (Nervous)

Chamomile   *Hydrastis*   *Valerian*   *Capsicum*

Earache

Mullein

Ear, running

Myrrh   *Echinacea*

Eczema

Myrrh   Bittersweet   Strawberry leaves   Dandelion
Burdock   Rhubarb

Emesis, to produce

Bayberry   *Lobelia*   *Boneset*   Bitter root

Emesis, to allay

Red Raspberry   Spearmint

Ear, Chronic discharge

Yellow dock   Mullein   *Echinacea*

Eruptive Diseases (acute)

Serpentaria   Pennyroyal   Scullcap   Pleurisy root
Chamomile

Eyes, sore

Eye Bright   Fennel

Eyes, sore—purulent

White Pond Lily

Fever (Influenza, LaGrippe)

Capsicum   *Lobelia*   Boneset   Pleurisy root   Scullcap

Fever (Malarial)

Barberry   Pleurisy root   *Capsicum*

Fever (Peritonitis)

Echinacea   *Lobelia*

Fever (Pneumonia)

Pleurisy root   Bonset   Motherwort   Feverfew
Ginger   Pennyroyal

Fever (Pleurisy)

Pleurisy root   Scullcap   Boneset   Ginger   Pennyroyal

Fever (Typhoid)

Geranium   Bayberry   *Echinacea*   Motherwort   *Passiflora*
Boneset   Pipsissewa

Fever (Scarlet)

Lobelia

Fever (Puerperal infection)

Echinacea   Feverfew   Myrrh

Fever (Smallpox)

Lobelia   Pennyroyal

Flatulence (wind colic)

Sweet flag   Catnip   Chamomile

Gangrenous Conditions

Echinacea   Myrrh

Gastritis (Chronic)

Bayberry   *Hydrastis*   *Chionanthus*   Sweet flag

Goitre

Bayberry   Oak Bark   Sea weed

Gout

Couch grass

Gall Stones

Chionanthus   Bitter root

Gravel

Couch grass   Corn silk   Shave grass   Knot grass
Buchu   Hemlock

Headache (Bilious)

Poplar Bark   *Chionanthus*   *Hydrastis*

Hard Drinkers, Remedies

Chionanthus   *Capsicum*   *Passiflora*   Feverfew

Headache (Chronic or Stomach)

Primrose   Motherwort

Headache (Nervous)

Cypripedium   *Pulsatilla*

Headache (Menstrual)

Pulsatilla   *Mitchella*

Headache (Sick, or Gastric)

Pulsatilla

Heart (weakness)

Scullcap   *Capsicum*   *Lobelia*   Cactus

Hemorrhages (nose, lungs, stomach and bowels)

Geranium   Shave grass   Witch hazel   Bayberry

Hemorrhages (Uterine)

Bayberry   Red raspberry   *Hydrastis*

Hysteria

Cypripedium   Scullcap   *Passiflora*   Pennyroyal   Tansy

Indigestion (Acute)

Lobelia   Poplar bark   *Hydrastis*   *Chionanthus*
Bitterroot   Dandelion

Indigestion (Atonic)

Hydrastis   Gentian   *Capsicum*   St. John's Wort

Indigestion (Flatulence and Eructions)

Feverfew   Calamus

Indigestion (Intestinal)

Hydrastis

Inflammation (Acute)

Witch hazel

Insomnia

Cypripedium   Scullcap   Motherwort   *Passiflora*

Jaundice

Chionanthus   Bitter root   Poplar bark   Feverfew
Barberry   Bitter herb   Couch grass

Jaundice (Gestation)

Chionanthus

Kidney

Motherwort   Corn silk   Juniper berries   Couch grass
Poplar bark   Shave grass

Kidney, Mucus

Motherwort   Linden flowers

Lactation, Aid to

Squaw vine   Milkwort

Leucorrhoea

Geranium   Hydrastis   Bayberry   Pulsatilla   Bearberry
Pond Lily   Sumac   Witch Hazel   Red Raspberry

Pipsissewa   Tormentil

Liver and Spleen

Barberry   Bitter herb   Dandelion   *Chionanthus   Ceanothus*

Liver (Acute Inflammation)

Chionanthus

Liver (Engorgement)

Dandelion

Liver (Dormant)

Motherwort   Bitter root   Dandelion

Liver (Torpid)

Hydrastis   Barberry   Gentian   Bitter herb
Bitter root   Rosemary

Lockjaw

Lobelia   Silverweed

Malassimilation

Bitter herb   *Chionanthus*   *Hydrastis*

Marasmus

Myrrh

Melancholy

Chamomile   *Cypripedium*   *Ceanothus*   *Pulsatilla*

Menstrual Irregularities

Chamomlle   *Cypripedium*   Scullcap   Squaw vine   Feverfew
Pulsatilla   Pennyroyal   Pipsissewa   Tansy

Mouth and Gums (sore)

Geranium   *Hydrastis*   Bayberry   *Echinacea*   Myrrh
Ceanothus   White Pond Lily

Nervine

Valerian   Scullcap   Lady Slipper   *Capsicum*
Hydrastis   Celery

Nervousness

Scullcap   Lady Slipper   Feverfew   *Passiflora*
Pulsatilla   Valerian

Neuralgia

Lady Slipper   *Pulsatilla*   Bitter root

Neuritis

Motherwort

Night Sweats

Geranium   Sage   Myrrh

Nipples (sore)

Squaw vine   Myrrh   Tannic acid

Nutrition and Blood Making

Bayberry   *Pulsatilla*   Lady Slipper

Parturition, made easy

Bayberry   Squaw vine   Feverfew

Poisonous Insects and Reptiles (bites)

Echinacea   *Lobelia*   Scullcap

Polypus (Nasal)

Geranium

Prostate (Enlarged)

Couch grass   *Chionanthus*   *Pulsatilla*   Pipsissewa

Pruritis

Witch hazel   Hemlock

Rectal (Ulceration)

Hydrastis

Respiratory (Congestion)

Lobelia   Pleurisy root

Rheumatism

Motherwort   Pipsissewa   Primrose   Couch grass
Bitter root   Burdock   *Macrotys*   Scurvy grass

Rheumatism (Articular)

Primrose   Motherwort

Rheumatism (Chronic)

Myrrh   Motherwort   Pipsissewa   Bitter root

Rheumatism (Gonorrhoeal)

Pipsissewa   Scurvy grass

Confinement (Rigid os)

Lobelia

Scrofula and Scurvy

Bayberry   *Echinacea*   Pipsissewa   Yellow Dock   Dandelion
Bitter root   Bitter sweet   Burdock   Sweet flag

Sexual Diseases (Gonorrhoea and Gleet)

Geranium root   *Hydrastis*   Poplar Bark   Bearberry
Hemlock   Scurvy grass   Tormentil

Sexual (Undue Excitement)

Scullcap   *Pulsatilla*

Sex Power (Increase)

Pulsatilla   Acorns   Oats

Sores and Wounds (Infected)

Echinacea   Myrrh

Spasms (Infantile)

Passiflora

Spermatorrhoea

Pulsatilla

Spleen

Ceanothus   Bayberry

Sprains, Bruises and Swellings

Chamomile   Myrrh

Spring (Remedy)

Rosemary   Rhubarb   Dandelion

Stomachic

Hydrastis   Gentian   *Capsicum*

Stomach (Bitters)

Hydrastis   *Anthemis*   *Berberis*   Rhubarb   *Capsicum*

Stomach (Debilitated)

Hydrastis   Chamomile

Stomach (Flaccid)

Bayberry   Gentian

Stomach (Worms)

Bitter herb

Syphilis

Barberry *Echinacea* *Ceanothus* Poplar bark
Bitter root Bitter sweet Yellow dock

Teething

Chamomile

Throat (Sore)

Bayberry Myrrh *Ceanothus* Mallow Flowers

Tonsilitis

Echinacea

Ulcers

Myrrh *Echinacea* *Calendula* Shave grass
Bittersweet ointment

Ulcers (Gastric)

Geranium *Hydrastis* Pleurisy root

Ulcers (Indolent)

Myrrh *Calendula*

Urine (Incontinence and Scaldy)

Couch grass Sumac Tansy Buchu Cleavers

Urine (Scanty and Painful)

Chionanthus Motherwort Corn silk Shave grass
Poplar bark Pipsissewa Hemlock Sumac
Red Raspberry Spearmint Burdock
Dandelion Cleavers

Uric Acid

Corn silk

Uterine (Dressings)

Calendula   *Hydrastis*   *Geranium*   Pond Lily

Uterus (Prolapsed)

Bayberry   Witch hazel

Uterine and Vaginal Ulceration

Hydrastis   *Calendula*   *Bearberry*   Pond Lily

Venereal Diseases (Chronic)

Geranium   *Hydrastis*   Couch grass   *Pulsatilla*   Poplar bark
Bearberry   Hemlock   Witch hazel   Red Raspberry
Burdock   Pipsissewa   Buchu   Cleavers
Scurvy grass   Tormentil

Vermifuge

Feverfew   Pumpkin seed

Vitalizer (Female)

Motherwort   *Pulsatilla*   *Mitchella*

Weakness (Female)

Geranium   Motherwort   *Mitchella*   *Pulsatilla*

Water Brash (Burning Eructions)

Sweet flag

Worms (Tape)

Male fern   Pumpkin seed

Youth (Culture)

Pulsatilla   Shave grass   Oat beards

GENERAL INDEX

225

41128